CANADIAN MEDICAL LIVES

J.C. BOILEAU GRANT

Anatomist Extraordinary

Clayton L.N. Robinson

Series Editor: T.P. Morley

Associated Medical Services, Incorporated
&
Fitzhenry & Whiteside
1993

Fithzenry & Whiteside
195 Allstate Parkway
Markham, Ontario L3R 4T8

Jacket design: Arne Roosman
Copy Editor: Frank English
Typesetting: Jay Tee Graphics Ltd.
Printing and Binding: Gagné Printing Ltd., Louiseville, Quebec, Canada

Fitzhenry & Whiteside wishes to acknowledge the generous assistance and ongoing support of **The Book Publishing Industry Development Programme** of the **Department of Communications, The Canada Council**, and **The Ontario Arts Council**.

Canadian Cataloguing in Publication Data

Robinson, Clayton (Clayton L. N.)
J.C. Boileau Grant

(Canadian medical lives : no. 14)
Includes bibliographical references and index.
ISBN 1-55041-149-7

1. Grant, J. C. Boileau (John Charles Boileau),
1886- . 2. Anatomists – Canada – Biography.
I. Hannah Institute for the History of Medicine.
II. Title. III. Series.

QM16.G73R6 1993 611′.0092 C93-094418-6

CANADIAN MEDICAL LIVES SERIES

The story of the Hannah Institute for the History of Medicine has been told by John B. Neilson and G.R. Paterson in *Associated Medical Services Incorporated: A History* (1987). Dr. Donald R. Wilson, President of AMS, and the Board of Directors decided that the Institute should produce this series of biographies as one of its undertakings.

The first ten biographies have now been published and can be obtained through the retail book trade or from Dundurn Press Ltd., 2181 Queen Street East, Suite 301, Toronto, Canada, M4E 1E5, and Dundurn Distribution, 73 Lime Walk, Headington, Oxford, England, OX3 7AD. The second group of biographies of which this is the second volume, can also be obtained through retail book stores or from the publisher, Fitzhenry and Whiteside.

J.C.Boileau Grant was one of two of the most renowned teachers of medicine in the English language; the other was his friend and colleague William Boyd. Each had the front-line practitioner in his sights. Grant's singleness of purpose was to bring up a generation of surgeons who knew exactly what they were doing once an operation had begun. His insistence on a sound grounding in topographic anatomy is today overshadowed by the demands of a more "scientific" approach to surgical practice—to the patient's peril. Doctors who as students came under Grant's spell in the dissecting room or library will be grateful to Clayton Robinson for keeping alive the memory of his teacher for the benefit of those who never knew him.

Future volumes include *R.M. Bucke* (Peter Rechnitzer), *William Henry Drummond* (J.B. Lyons) and *William Beaumont* (Julian Smith).

There is no shortage of meritorious subjects. Willing and capable authors are harder to acquire. The Institute is therefore deeply grateful to authors who have committed their time and skill to the series.

T.P. Morley
Series Editor
1993

CANADIAN MEDICAL LIVES SERIES

Duncan Graham by Robert B. Kerr and Douglas Waugh

Bill Mustard by Marilyn Dunlop

Joe Doupe by Terence Moore

Emily Stowe by Mary Beacock Fryer

Clarence Hincks by Charles G. Roland

Francis A.C. Scringer, V.C., by Suzanne Kingsmill

Earle P. Scarlett by F.W. Musselwhite

R.G. Ferguson by C. Stuart Houston

Harold Griffith by Richard Bodman and Deirdre Gillies

Maude Abbott by Douglas Waugh

William Boyd by Ian Carr

J.C.Boileau Grant by C.L.N. Robinson

CONTENTS

Acknowledgements

The sources of this biography are many: a teacher at the Collegiate and Vocational school in Renfrew, Ontario; an anatomy professor at Queen's University; the Navy, especially the Royal Navy; Professor Dermid L.C. Bingham, Professor of Surgery at Queen's; Dr. J.C.B. Grant himself at the University of Toronto; the University of Saskatchewan at Saskatoon; and the late Dr. David Christie and his late widow, Alice, in Vancouver.

To begin at the beginning. At my high school in Renfrew, Miss Catherine O'Brien was a classics teacher. It was she who sowed the seed in my mind that I might be good enough to take up a profession. I was suspicious of law, but I became attracted to the idea of medicine as a career and as a teenager I resolved to pursue it.

Miss O'Brien was one of those heaven-sent teachers who became foster-mother to me and to other pupils. She lived to be ninety. Whenever I visited her, which was about once a year in her later life, and invited her out to dinner, there always seemed to be a rush of other former students who wanted to honour her as well. Miss O'Brien was the attraction, not the returning wanderer. It is to her I owe my enjoyment of literature.

In the medical faculty at Queen's University there were many fine teachers. A stand-out was our professor of anatomy, Dr. Donald C. Matheson. He was a "Mr. Chips" of a teacher. We all referred to him as "Mattie". He was a bachelor and lived with his unmarried sister. He knew the first name of every student and he would likely have wanted to address them so, but it was not done in those days, and in any case he would have been too shy. Dr. Matheson taught from Cunningham's textbook, while we used the Cunningham dissecting manual. We also used Gray's textbook. Jamieson's ("Wee Jamie") loose-leaf highly coloured anatomical diagrams (*Illustrations of Regional Anatomy*) were much regarded too. Dr. J.C.B. Grant's *A Method of Anatomy* was already published, but was not immediately popular, and probably had not yet been recommended. It was Mattie who made the study of gross anatomy interesting, so important to an aspiring surgeon.

When Matheson retired at the usual age of sixty-five from Queen's he worked as a gardener for a medical colleague for five years. It so happened that at the University of Saskatchewan at Saskatoon the professor of anatomy, Dr. Altschul, died suddenly and Saskatoon needed a teacher to take his place. Mattie, in excellent health from his five years out of doors, was contacted and offered the position, which he accepted. This was during the time I was in the Surgery Department, when I frequently had lunch with "Mattie". I even gave a lecture on the applied anatomy of the thorax once, with Dr. Matheson sitting like a guardian Buddha in the back row. Like that other inspired teacher, Dr. Grant, Matheson came out of retirement to teach again, this time for another five years.

When I returned to Canada from active service in the Far East I took a temporary hospital job in pathology in Kingston. I asked the newly appointed Professor in Surgery at Queen's, Dr. Dermid Bingham, about training for surgery in Canada. Dr. Bingham was an Edinburgh graduate, had trained in Britain, and had been a surgical specialist in the Royal Army Medical Corps during the War. Dr. Bingham replied: "I cannot help you here, for I have just arrived and do not know many Canadian surgeons. But, if you wanted to go to England, I could give you a leg up with Professor Aird at the British Postgraduate Medical School, or Rodney Smith at St. George's Hospital. Of course, if you go there for postgraduate work, you would have to do the English Fellowship."

I welcomed this advice and thought immediately about doing a year first as a demonstrator in anatomy, in preparation for the first part of the English fellowship exam. The two demonstrator positions in Kingston had been filled by Dr. Matheson. So I wrote to Dr. Grant at Toronto and asked for an appointment in his department. He gave me a place, "sight unseen". It was now near the beginning of the academic year, so I moved to Toronto and found a bed-sitting room near the University. I met Dr. Grant and very quickly liked him, notwithstanding the awe he inspired in me.

Grant's *A Method of Anatomy* and its companion, *Atlas of Anatomy*, were, of course, the standard texts in the department. When I took my first cursory look into the *Method,* I thought it lacked detail. But after studying from it and teaching with it I realized it had *everything* in it. The reasoning was flawless and every fact seemed simplified. After the year in Grant's department, the primary examination (at least in anatomy) held few fears for me and I sailed to England to face the examiners at the Royal College of Surgeons and passed. Clinical experience in London, with guidance from Professor Aird, followed and, with success at the final examination, my anxieties were laid to rest. On my return to Canada I joined the surgical staff at the University of Saskatchewan, moving later to the University of British Columbia in Vancouver.

My elder brother, Dr. Cecil Robinson, had been practising in Vancouver as an internal medicine and rheumatology specialist. One of his patients, Dr. David Christie, also an internal medicine specialist, was the brother of Dr. Grant's wife, Catriona (and of Enid, the wife of a fellow Scot, Dr. William Boyd). When my brother was out of Vancouver he would ask me to "pinch hit" for him by keeping an eye on Dr. Christie.

David Christie kept enlarged photographs of Dr. Grant and Dr. Boyd in his bedroom. I would chat with him about his famous brothers-in-law during my visits. When he died, his widow, Alice, gave me several books and other valuable memorabilia that Dr. Grant had handed to David. One item was a detailed *curriculum vitae* that Dr. Grant had typed at the age of seventy-three.

In those ten typewritten pages were facts that I and many others, even at the University of Toronto, had not known: his magnificent record in World War I and the Boileau link on his mother's side, for example. Based on some of this material I wrote a short appreciation of Dr. Grant for the *Canadian Journal of Surgery.*[1] On account of this article, the Hannah Institute for the History of Medicine in Toronto contacted me to ask if I would write a biography as I ''seemed to know the family''. I wasted no time in accepting the honour.

It is fairly easy to describe the purely professional aspects of a man's life; it amounts to little more than an expanded *curriculum vitae* but it does not reveal the whole man. The many aspects of Dr. Grant's personal side which I recount have largely been given to me by nieces and nephews on the Grant side, and by nieces on the Christie side. A brother of Catriona, Archie Christie, who has lived and worked in England for most of his life but who visits Canada annually to look after the family estates, has been most helpful.

It is a pleasure to acknowledge many other sources of information and the encouragement and support given by numerous people. High on the list are the family members who have written detailed letters, sent pamphlets written by forbears and ancestors and unearthed family photographs. The last include not only individual pictures, but also whole sections of a family album. Such trust!

On the Grant side, two children of Dr. Grant's elder sister, Nellie, Mrs. Alison (Reid) Lofting, who resides in Nottingham, England, and Ian Reid, a retired classics school teacher, who now lives in Dundas, Ontario, have given more help than can be put into words. Ian supplied the greater part of the Grant family tree; his sister, Alison, added notes and filled in some gaps. Mrs. Mary (Molly) Kolsky, of Providence, Rhode Island, has also been helpful with information from her uncle (though much younger than she) Travers Grant, a son of John Charles Grant by his second marriage, and from Robin McGibbon, her cousin.

On the Christie side there are several who have sent abundant information: Mrs. Cleone Stoloff, a daughter of the late Mrs. Mary Feir, the eldest Christie sister, from Portland, Oregon, has supplied the Boileau family tree; Archie Christie, the only surviving Christie brother; Fleming and Ben McConnell, sons of the late Isobel Christie, a younger sister of Catriona and Enid Christie.

Professor Audrey Kerr, Head of the Faculty of Medicine Library at the University of Manitoba, has given unending help. The archivist of the medical faculty of the University of Toronto has supplied much information.

For recollections of Grant, I am indebted to many of his students and colleagues, including Dr. John Hamilton, at one time Professor of Pathology and Dean of Medicine, Toronto; Professor Neil Watters of the Department of Surgery, Toronto; Dr. W.D. Stevenson, retired head of neurosurgery at Dalhousie University, Halifax; Dr. Robert J. Cowan, class of 1941, and former head of plastic surgery, University of British Columbia; and Dr. J.W. Kalkman, class of 1959, now of the Department of Anaesthesia, St. Paul's Hospital, Vancouver. Dr. Hertz Rotenberg identified almost all the Demonstrators surrounding Grant in one of the illustrations no one else could do it!

Dr. Michael Alms, a graduate of Bristol University, an orthopaedic surgeon and my long-time friend and colleague, has indoctrinated me into the intricacies of a word processor and gave me a program on touch typing. Mrs. Teresa (Jackson) Carbonneau, now a Vancouver resident, a daughter of a former "Chief" of mine in England, has held my hand with the word processor and is able to "command" it when it misbehaves.

Dr. James Sandilands in Vancouver put me in touch with William Small, his former shipmate in the RNVR, now a retired surgeon in Edinburgh, who has produced a great deal of information about Loanhead and Grantown-on-Spey.

I also thank Dr. Fritz Baumgartner, a graduate of UCLA, who provided me with anecdotes from his university and brought me up to date on the career of Dr. R.J.Last.

A former fellow house surgeon from the Hammersmith days, Dr. Sita (Achaya) Iyappa, has filled in details about Professor Last and Dr. Grant. Sita became Professor of Anatomy at the Lady Harding Medical College in New Delhi and then Dean of Medicine at that college. She recently informed me that a fairly new college in Bombay has been named after Dr. Grant: The Grant Medical College.

My brother-in-law in London, England, Dr. Peter Purves, formerly head of the Section on Whales and Porpoises at the British Museum, has laboured at the British Library to look up details of the Boileau and Grant families.

Karen MacCougan, Canadian National Exhibition Archives, kindly provided the photograph of the Lord Stanley whom Grant rescued in World War I.

Various colleagues and associates at the Vancouver General Hospital had the patience to listen to my travails of authorship. Dr. Peter Allen especially deserves much praise.

Dr. Norman Rigby, a long-time friend, has given me support in many ways. As a member of the Board of the Eric Hamber Foundation in Vancouver, he has solicited the Foundation's interest in this biography. Brigadier J.S. Ryder of the Ministry of Defence at Stanmore, Middlesex, kindly gave me the information about the Military Cross and bar won by each of those valiant Grant brothers, J.C.B. and Allan.

Sister Teresa Kergoat of St. Vincent's Hospital (now known as St. Vincent's Health Care Society) helped me with a letter in French to the office of the Mayor of Paris, Jacques Chiraud. This was when I first started to trace the Boileau family tree. The archive department replied with regret that they did not keep records as far back as 1255.

Mrs. Sheila Swanson, head librarian of the Toronto Academy of Medicine, kindly produced the 1642 engraving of Wirsung's dissection of the pancreatic ducts which had been presented to the Academy by Dr. Grant. Mr. Harry Fancy, Curator, and Ms. Val Hepworth, Assistant Curator of the Whitehaven Museum, Cumbria, England, and Miss Anne Dick of the Daniel Hay Library in Whitehaven, all sacrificed a working day to the procurement of the engraving of the Whitehaven Infirmary and the evidence of Grant's appointment as House Surgeon.

Finally, thanks are owed to my children, Moya, Richard and Elspeth, who forgave their father's neglect; and to my wife, Kathleen, who has had the forbearance to remain alone when I was in my garret, struggling to do justice to the memory of John Charles Boileau Grant.

Chapter 1

Anatomical Analogies

THE ELEVENTH edition of Dr. Grant's *A Method of Anatomy* was published in April 1989. It was edited by Dr. Charles Slonecker, Professor and Head of Anatomy at the University of British Columbia, and by Dr. John Basmajian, now Professor Emeritus in Anatomy and Medicine at McMaster University, who had been head of anatomy at Toronto and at Queen's University at Kingston, Ontario.

In earlier decades, anatomy and physiology were the bastions of the student's curriculum for the first two years of medical school. A knowledge of topographic, that is, gross anatomy was the foundation of all surgery and much of internal medicine. Many of the country's surgeons built their skill on the foundation of Grant's teaching, in person or from his textbook.

A Method of Anatomy is widely used. It is perhaps not quite as popular as *Gray's Anatomy* which is now in its fortieth edition. In the foreword to *Gray's Anatomy*, Dr. John Crocco of St. Vincent's Hospital, New York, states, "Gray's book will probably be the premier text in Anatomy over the next 100 years. Gray's book will be remembered by twentieth century physicians as the Anatomy text of our age." If, as most students would agree, illustrations are as important as text in a book on anatomy, then this statement is open to question. In the

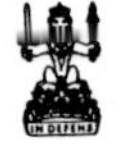

1861 – 1965

025263

Extract of an entry in a REGISTER of BIRTHS

Registration of Births, Deaths and Marriages (Scotland) Act 1965

No.	1 Name and surname	2 When and where born	3 Sex	4 Name, surname, and rank or profession of father Name, and maiden surname of mother Date and place of marriage	5 Signature and qualification of informant, and residence, if out of the house in which the birth occurred	6 When and where registered and signature of registrar
101	John Charles Boileau GRANT	1886 February Sixth 7h 30m am Free Church Manse Loanhead Lasswade	M	John Charles Grant Free Church Minister Ellen Jemima Grant m.s. Clarke 1883 June 28 Islington London	*Signed* John Charles Grant Father present	1886 April 2nd At Lasswade *Signed* Wm Brunton *Registrar*

The above particulars are extracted from a Register of Births for the Parish of Lasswade

in the County of Edinburgh

Given under the Seal of the General Register Office, New Register House, Edinburgh, on 15th August 1988

The above particulars incorporate any subsequent corrections or amendments to the original entry made with the authority of the Registrar General.

Warning

It is an offence under section 53(3) of the Registration of Births, Deaths and Marriages (Scotland) Act 1965 for any person to pass as genuine any copy or reproduction of this extract which has not been made by the General Register Office and authenticated by the Seal of that Office.

Any person who falsifies or forges any of the particulars on this extract or knowingly uses, gives or sends as genuine any false or forged extract is liable to prosecution under section 53(1) of the said Act.

RXB 5(T)

Copy of Grant's birth certificate.

recent paperback edition the drawings are limited and only a few are in colour.

Dr. Grant's *Atlas of Anatomy*, on the other hand, is the most popular book of anatomical illustrations in use today in the English-speaking world. The ninth edition, published by the University of Toronto Press, has sold over 50,000 copies. His practical manual, the *Dissector*, is also used widely.

When Grant described in his lectures an anatomical structure—a nerve, for example—he would say, "It has a beginning, an end, and a middle. It's like the Trans-Canada Highway. That highway begins in St. John's, Newfoundland, and ends in Victoria, British Columbia. At each end it has a body of water, the Cabot Strait at the east, and the Georgia Strait at the west. In the middle it crosses the maritime provinces of Nova Scotia and New Brunswick, the industrial provinces of Quebec and Ontario, the three prairie provinces, and then mountainous British Columbia."

The analogy stood the student in good stead for the searching test of the primary examination in anatomy for the Fellowship of the Royal College of Surgeons of England. The laconic command, "Describe the 7th cranial nerve," is more easily obeyed by following Grant's method, particularly in the case of a nerve with such a complicated course as it passes out of the skull. It's also not a bad analogy of Grant's life.

Grant's beginning was in Loanhead, near Edinburgh, where he was born on 6 February 1886. His ending was in the Toronto General Hospital on 14 August 1973 eighty-seven years later. Between these events, his life, like the course of the seventh cranial nerve, was complicated but purposeful.

He attended the Royal High School, Edinburgh, until 1895, when his family moved to Nottingham, England. There he enrolled in the Boys' High School and attended it until 1902, after which he spent a year at school in Grantown-on-Spey, Scotland. He studied Medicine at the University of Edinburgh from 1903 till 1908, graduating with second class honours. After graduation he obtained an appointment as the only resident house officer at the Infirmary, Whitehaven, Cumberland.

Whitehaven owed its importance to the industrial revolution as a coal-mining town and busy port on the Irish Sea. The families of the Earls of Lonsdale had dominated the community since the seventeenth

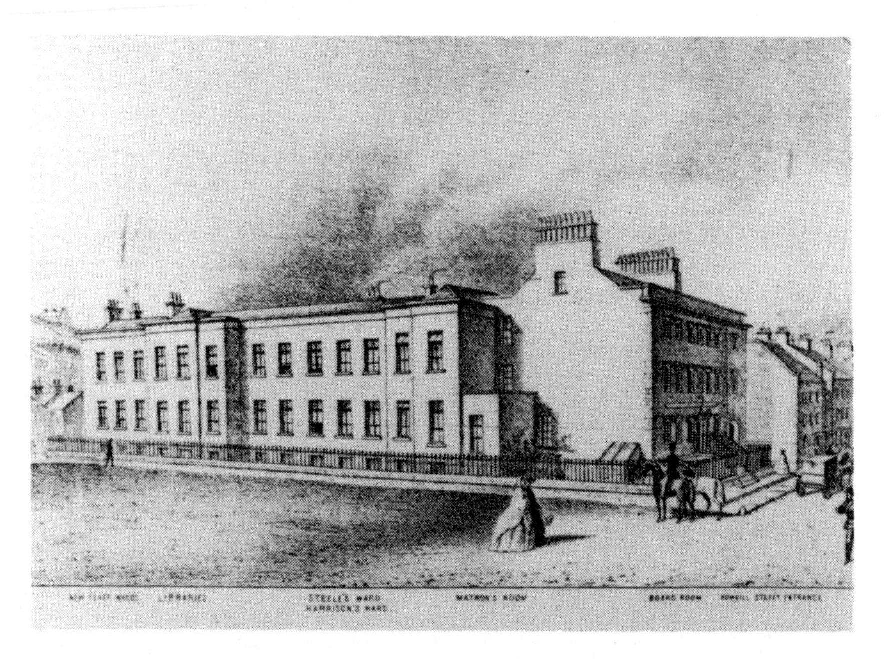

Whitehaven and West Cumberland Infirmary as it still appeared in Grant's time as House Surgeon (from Document 12 in Sickness and Poverty in XIX Century Whitehaven. *Courtesy Whitehaven Museum)*

century, holding their position up to the end of the nineteenth century by ownership of the extensive coal mines. The Lonsdales had always been prominent in the construction and management of the town's institutions, including the public Infirmary. A private home had been bought in 1829 and enlarged into the Whitehaven and West Cumberland Infirmary with 59 beds.[1] In 1924 it was moved to Lonsdale Castle, a residential extravaganza, which by then had become a burden to the family fortune.

Grant was the only resident doctor at the Infirmary. His responsibility was to look after the patients as directed by the handful of practitioners appointed to the hospital by the trustees. The attending staff of local general practitioners, according to the universal staffing arrangement of public hospitals of the time, was unpaid and its members performed all the surgical operations. The salary Grant received is not known, but an earlier house surgeon forfeited his appointment because he rejected a salary of "81 pound per annum, with taxes, coals and candles, the appointment to last for three years". The next house surgeon, however, benifited from the recalcitrance of his predecessor to the tune of £100 a year.

Since the Infirmary was for the benefit of the working man and his family, it was decided in 1907 (the year before Grant's arrival) at the Annual General Meeting that "each company of workmen in the surrounding neighbourhood that subscribed Five Guineas per annum to the Infirmary should be allowed a representative on the General Committee." The added representation "proved to be of great advantage to all concerned"[2] and, perhaps, to the house surgeon's pocket.

Much of the work at the Infirmary was of a surgical nature, with the injured from the mines and other industrial installations occupying most of the beds. Indeed the resident doctor was appointed as house surgeon rather than house physician, and the attending medical staff members were referred to in the hospital records as "Honorary Surgeons" although they were general practitioners. In the community of 19,320, remote from a medical school, every medical practitioner was "general" without specialty pretensions.

From 1909 to 1911 Grant demonstrated anatomy in the University of Edinburgh under the renowned Dr. Cunningham, and from 1911 to 1913 in the University of Durham, at Newcastle-on-Tyne, under Professor R. Howden who was then the editor of *Gray's Anatomy*. In

1913 Grant moved to the Infirmary at Bristol as resident medical officer in the Ear, Nose and Throat Department. In those days a few medical graduates were marked out for house officer appointments in the teaching hospital of their alma mater. The rest had to fend for themselves. There were no organized training programs in the modern sense. Grant's house appointments at Whitehaven and Bristol lent no prestige to his name, but they gave him a little money (by contrast, the teaching hospital appointments were virtually unpaid) and a lot of experience.

When Great Britain declared war on Germany on 4 August 1914, Grant volunteered immediately. He received his commission in the Royal Army Medical Corps on 2 November 1914. His army attachments as regimental medical officer included the Grenadier Guards and the 8th Battalion, Black Watch (Royal Highlanders). He was later posted to the 58th Casualty Clearing Station as an ear, nose and throat surgeon. He was mentioned in despatches in September 1916; he received the Military Cross (immediate award) in September 1917, and a bar to the Military Cross (immediate award) on 19 August 1918 (2nd Army).

Shortly after he was demobilized he was invited to be Professor of Anatomy in the University of Manitoba in Winnipeg and arrived there on 21 October 1919. Grant remained in Winnipeg until 1930, when he accepted the Chair of Anatomy at the University of Toronto. He held this position until his retirement in 1956, when he was appointed Curator of the Anatomy Museum in the University. But his academic life did not come to an end at that time.

In 1961 he was invited as the Visiting Professor of Anatomy in the University of California at Los Angeles where he taught for another ten years. In his second year there, he was so highly regarded by the students that they dedicated to him their annual medical year book, *Meducla*.

His final years in Toronto were bedevilled by cancer. In 1971 he developed a tumour just below the larynx which was treated by radiation at the Princess Margaret Hospital. Within a year another tumour developed in the trachea, but he decided to forego further treatment. Refusing all feeding, he resolutely turned toward the wall and in two days quietly died. Thus the thread of his life ended. St Paul's valediction to Timothy can as well apply to J.C. Boileau Grant, the last of the great topographic anatomists:

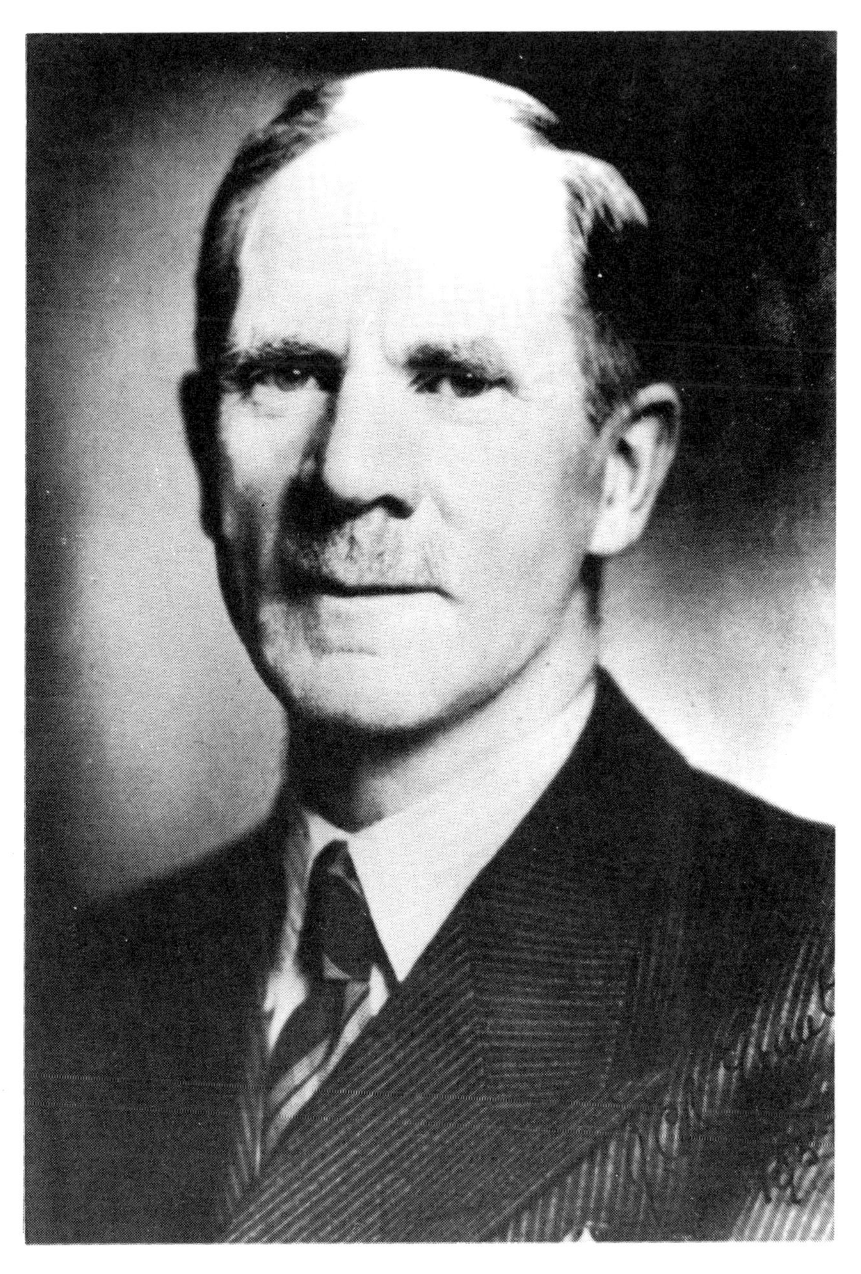

Professor J.C.B. Grant at the time of his official retirement, University of Toronto, 1956.

I have fought a good fight,
I have finished my course,
I have kept the faith.
II Timothy. 4,7.

— Chapter 2 —

Forebears

IN HIS *curriculum vitae,* Dr. Grant says:

> I, John Charles Boileau Grant, was born on 6th February, 1886, at Loanhead, six miles from Edinburgh, where my father was a Presbyterian minister. My paternal grandfather, John Grant, leased a farm at Grantown-on-Spey, Morayshire, Scotland, from the local landlord, the Earl of Seafield, and he was in possession of a receipt showing that his forebears had leased it since the year 1630. My mother was a direct descendant, 20th generation, of Etienne Boileau who was the first Mayor or Provost of Paris, in the year 1255. Being of the Reformed Church (Huguenots), some of the Boileaus left France for England and Ireland in the year 1685.

Grant's matter-of-fact statement about the Boileau ancestry hardly does justice to the sufferings of the Huguenots which the Edict of Nantes (1598) was supposed to end. The Edict, promulgated to assure the reformers freedom from persecution, was persistently opposed by the clergy with every administrative and legal means in their power. Reformed churches were demolished and their Protestant members deprived of their civil freedom, property and liberty of conscience. Under the influence of torture, they foreswore their religious beliefs and espoused Roman Catholicism. At last, in 1685, capitulating to unrelenting pressure from the church, Louis XIV revoked the Edict of Nantes and legalized what had in fact already been achieved, the suppression of the Reform Movement.

A part of the Boileau line survived the Massacre of St. Bartholomew and subsequent pogroms in France calculated to eliminate the Huguenots. Maurice Boileau, one must assume, reverted under pressure to the established church since he kept the family titles and retained the estates. Another Boileau, Charles, in the year of revocation of the Edict of Nantes, refusing to surrender his beliefs, joined the hundreds of thousands who had forsaken the country which now no longer gave even a pretence of protection to religious dissidents. Many fled to Prussia and other continental sanctuaries; as many, like Charles, sailed for England. There he sired several children, only two of whom survived to adulthood: a daughter and a son, Simon, who carried on the family name. (For more details of the Boileau line, please see Appendix 2.)

The 1885 edition of *Groome's Gazeteer* has the following information about the Loanhead of Grant's childhood:

> It has charming environs, including a very romantic reach of the North Esk's glen; it mainly consists of two streets, which join each other at an obtuse angle; and it contains a number of good houses, which serve as a summer retreat for some of the Edinburgh townsfolk, though its own population consists in great measure of miners and those engaged in the oil-works and paper-mills. It has a post office, with money order, savings bank, insurance and telegraph departments, a branch of the British Linen Company's Bank, a water supply by pipes, a police station, public and R.C. schools, and a bowling club. It became a police burgh in 1884, and is governed by a provost, 2 bailies, and 6 commissioners. Places of worship are an Established church, a Free church, a Reformed Presbyterian church, a Primitive Methodist chapel, and St. Margaret's Roman Catholic church. Loanhead Quoad Sacra church is in the presbytery of Dalkeith and synod of Lothian and Twee-

dale. Minister's stipend 223 pounds sterling. Population of burgh 2493 (1881), 3244 (1891).

In recent years, when coal is not so necessary as a source of heat and power, the coal slag heaps have been cleaned up. The slag is being used for roadbeds and such.[1]

Grant's great-grandfather, Donald Grant, was the last of seven or eight generations to farm at Lagg, about four miles northeast of Grantown. In 1828, on the death of his ninety-seven-year-old father, Capt. Alex Grant, the headship of the Tullochgorm Grants nominally passed to Donald, but he never claimed it. After Donald's death, Lagg was used as a summer resort by his son John and family after they had moved to Grantown.

This John was Dr. Grant's grandfather (1822-1882). He had started law studies at Edinburgh, but gave them up at the age of nineteen when his father died. He became an "accountant, auctioneer and valuator", and took up residence in Grantown.

John Grant followed his father's interest in supporting the disrupting of the Church of Scotland in 1843, and succeeded, against considerable opposition, in establishing the Free Church in Grantown.

Although John Grant spoke Gaelic he did not encourage his family to speak it. He was a Liberal and was election manager in 1865 for Sir George Macpherson Grant of Ballindalloch who unsuccessfully challenged the conservative establishment in Strathspey. In those days voting was open, not secret, and few would have opposed the political views of their landlord, Grant of Feuchie. Lady Seafield was particularly vindictive towards John Grant. As punishment for his political activities, the Seafields deprived John Grant of his Lagg farm. Macpherson Grant of Ballindalloch offered him one of his best farms, Lagmore, in its place but John declined it. About 1845, he married a widow, Jane Campbell (née Shaw), who was his senior by about ten years. She already had three daughters, and bore four more daughters and two sons. John Charles, who would become the father of Dr. Grant, was the eldest in this second family.

J.C.B.Grant's father was raised in Strathspey. He studied at the University and Free Church College, Aberdeen. After an indentured year at Laven, he was ordained at Loanhead in 1880. In 1883 he married Ellen J. Clarke and they moved to Nottingham in 1895. Meanwhile the Free Church congregation at Loanhead, as elsewhere in Scotland, joined with the United Presbyterian Church in 1900 to form the United Free Church. In 1929 it in turn united with the established Church of Scotland.

The Rev. John Charles Grant (1854-1942) was paid a fine tribute when he retired from his Presbyterian church, Belgrave Square in Nottingham. It was said he was undaunted in the early, difficult years of his ministry there, and that Grant (a corruption of the Norman *Le Grande*) was a most fitting name. Tall, erect, of good carriage, his was a presence to be remembered.

John Charles, like his father, espoused the cause of the poor crofters, and was "at outs" with the landed class. He was a champion for any cause where injustice was perceived. Some of his fighting spirit may have come from his grandmother who was a daughter of General Wright, a follower of "Bonnie Prince Charlie". During his university career at Aberdeen John Charles was friendly with many great men. After his ordination at Loanhead in 1880 he received his first ministerial "call" to nearby Laven where he was privileged to meet many distinguished people of his day.

One of these was Dr. John Balfour, uncle of Robert Louis Stevenson. Another was Mr. Buchan, father of Lord Tweedsmuir—the future writer and Governor General of Canada, then but a little boy.

At the end of a year at Laven when he became a licensed minister of the church there occurred an incident typical of his independent attitude. When asked to sign the Confession of Faith he did so "with reservations". Asked what they were, he said, "Well, you all have them," and went on to say that he "did not believe that God made all things in six days."

"But does not the Bible say so?" he was asked.

"No!" he replied. "I think not. The Confession takes the Hebrew allegory and makes it a matter of fact."

His questioner turned aside and said, "Moderator, give Mr. Grant the pen. He is the most orthodox man here." His courage had served him well.

Rev. Grant gathered around him a considerable body of young men and he did his utmost to direct their thoughts and energies along wise lines. His sermons were literary treats, inspired and popular. Alas, some of his most promising admirers met their end in the battlefields of Flanders.

After his death a stained-glass window was placed in the church in his memory. It was a picture of the Apostle Paul, whom he so often quoted. He holds a book which represents his Epistles, and bears a sword signifying the Good Fight. Palm trees in the background are an allusion to the victory of which they are the symbol. The window bears the inscription STAND FAST, appropriate for a Grant whose battle cry is "Stand Fast Craigellachie."

On the Sunday of the dedication of the window, his grandson, Ian Reid, read the lesson. Mrs. Reid, the Rev. Grant's eldest daughter, unveiled the window in the presence of many members of the Grant family, his grandchildren and great-grandchildren.

Rev. John Charles Grant wrote his personal reminiscences, *A Humble Human*, which were never published.[2] He recounted his own boyhood in Strathspey and his later career, but almost completely omitted any reference to his family, an omission prompted, perhaps, by the dour conviction that his family was as unworthy as himself for special mention! After his retirement he did write *Letters from the Mountains*[3] apparently in response to his son John's interest in his family background in Scotland. To satisfy the request he dealt with the history of Strathspey and the Grants.

John Charles Grant married Ellen Jemima Clarke (1859-1900) in 1883, in Islington, London. They had nine children, five boys and four girls. Ellen died in childbirth with the ninth child on 1 January 1900. The baby, who lived for only a few hours, was named Benoni, Hebrew for Benjamin, "child of my sorrow". From his professional knowledge of Hebrew, John Charles would have chosen the baby's name to mark the poignancy of his twofold loss.

The eldest girl, Ellen (usually called Nellie), was then sixteen and had to leave school to bring up her seven brothers and sisters. The youngest children knew as their mother only Nellie, who also had to act as the minister's wife for social functions.

In 1924 Rev. J.C.Grant, now aged seventy, married Susan Macy. They had a son, Charles Baring Travers, born on 25 January 1925. After completing his National Service in the Royal Navy and acquiring a degree at Oxford, he decided to take up medicine. He graduated from St. Bartholomew's Hospital in 1956 and is still in general practice at Horsham in Sussex.

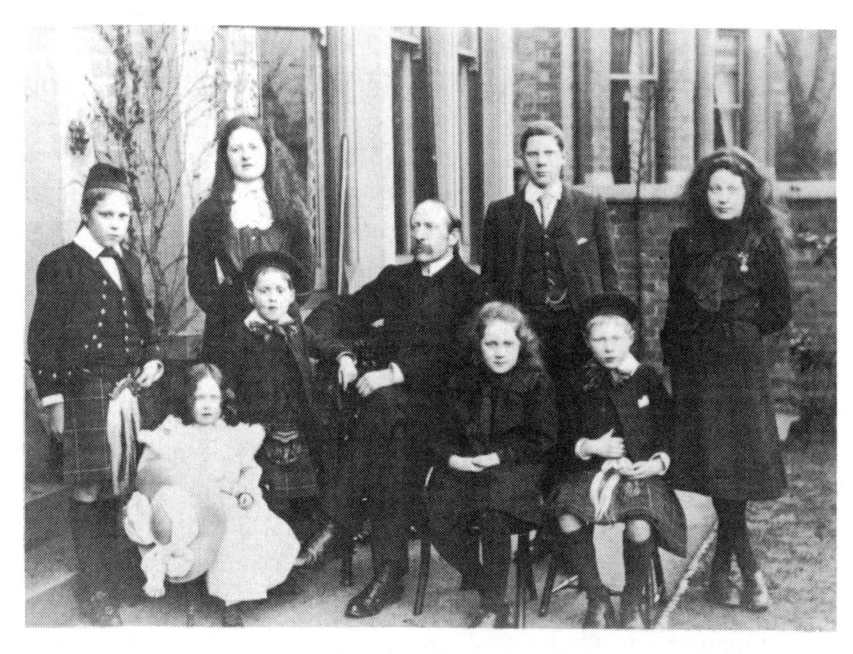

The Grant family, outside the Manse, 16 Baker Street, Nottingham, about 1900, probably at the time of Mrs. Grant's death. Standing: Donald, Ellen ("Nellie"), J.C.B., Mary ("Poppy"). Front: Grace ("Grizel"), Allan, Reverend John Charles, Dorothy, Louis (Ludovic). J.C.B. has graduated from the stigma (in Nottingham) of the kilt.

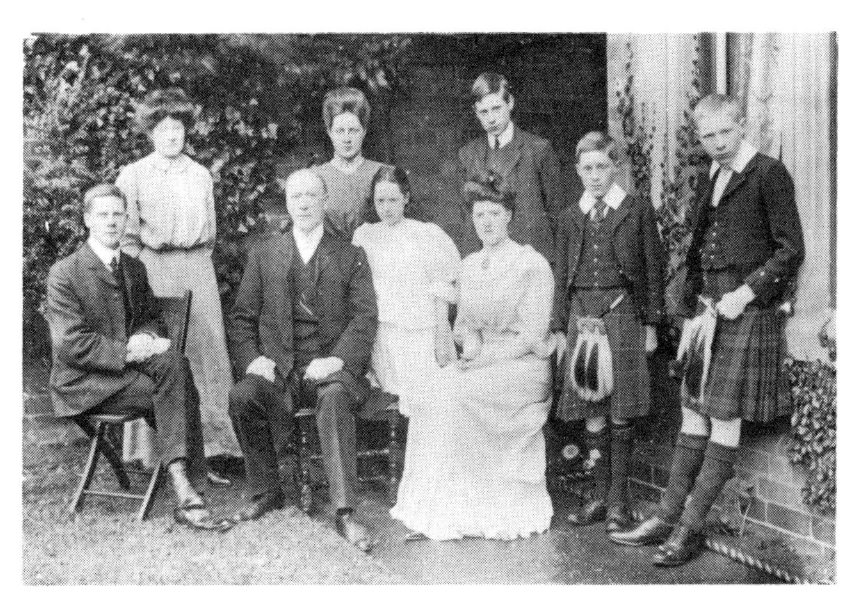

The Grant family, outside the Manse, 16 Baker Street, Nottingham, about 1907. Back row, standing: Mary ("Poppy"), Dorothy, Donald, Allan, Louis. Sitting: J.C.B., Rev. J.C. Grant, Grace ("Grizel"), Ellen ("Nellie").

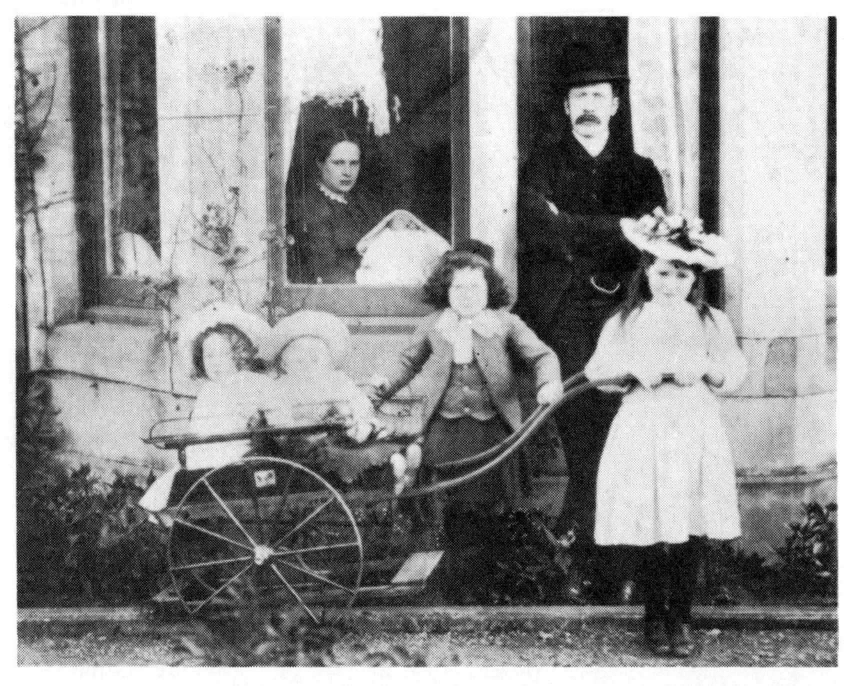

Loanhead, circa 1890. Rev. John and Ellen with baby Louis (?) in her arms. In front: ''Poppy'' and Donald (?), in the cart; J.C.B. (age 4-5) and Nellie standing. J.C.B is wearing traditional Scottish clothes that go with the kilt. This is the only surviving picture of Ellen (J.C.B.'s mother).

Ian Reid recalls his grandfather:

I find it difficult to assess the true relationship of this large family with their father, the Rev. John Charles; it was a matter never really discussed by my mother. My own impressions are that their attitude to him was one of dutiful respect, perhaps tinged with awe. He certainly had a domineering personality, and a six-foot upright body to match it. I remember what an impressive figure he presented on Sundays as he strode from the Manse to the Church, about a mile away, wearing frock coat and top hat. I also remember that when we children went to a meal at the Manse, we were not expected to talk unless first addressed by an adult. But he certainly had a softer side to his character, and he loved a good joke. He was greatly loved, as well as respected, by members of his congregation; they showed their gratitude by paying for his trip to Canada in 1922 at the time of his son John's marriage.

He was a good preacher, but not an intolerant bible-thumper. He had the ability to think for himself and the courage to speak his thoughts, however unpopular they might be. He was also well known in Nottingham for his social work, notably with actors and entertainers visiting the city who stayed in cheap lodgings near the Theatre Royal and the Empire Music Hall, not far from the church.

Some of the Rev. Grant's strength of character must have rubbed off on his children but, I think, not so much of his religion. My mother was a devoted church attender and worker, but she declined invitations to be an Elder of the church. His son John, to the best of my knowledge, had no allegiance to any church in Canada. I suspect that he was an open-minded agnostic, but I cannot be sure about this.

Practically nothing has been written about Dr. Grant's mother, Ellen (née Clarke). Her physical characteristics and personality have not been related by or passed on to any of her grandchildren nor by Dr. Grant himself. The only surviving photograph was taken through a window with five young children, one a baby in her arms. It must have been at Loanhead, for "Dr. John" appears to be four or five years old, with a full head of curly hair and wearing a kilt. Mrs. Grant has long hair parted in the middle and tied in a bun. Her fine features reflect a determination necessary for the successful raising of a large family on a minister's stipend. She had taught the two oldest children, Nellie and John, at home before they were old enough to travel by themselves to the day school in Edinburgh. This was before the family moved to Nottingham.

Ellen was a daughter of James Boileau Clarke (b. 1832) and Elizabeth Ramsay; she had two younger sisters and a brother. Her paternal grandfather, Dr. James Clarke, had married Harriet Ann Boileau, a daughter of Simeon Peter Boileau and Hannah Ribton de Renzey, his wife.

Mrs. Alison (Reid) Lofting writes of the Grant clan:

> There is a drop of Huguenot Boileau blood in the family through the Rev. John Charles Grant's first wife, Ellen Clarke, but the Grant clan has an even more interesting history. It goes back to 1066 when William the Conqueror came to England from Normandy. The Normans were not Latin French but were originally Norsemen from Scandinavia. This may account for our family's red or fair hair and blue eyes, and their tall, manly bearing. In Normandy the name was originally Grante, meaning grand or tall. In Normandy the family motto was ''*Tenons Ferme*'', the same as the motto of the Scottish clan Grant, ''*Stand Fast*''. The new Grant settlers in England seem to have been granted land in the midlands — Nottinghamshire and Lincolnshire — where there are still place names such as Grantham and Granby. The legend is that one of the Grants was caught poaching in the King's forest and as punishment, for this crime was vicious, he escaped to Scotland.
>
> The first record of the name Grant in Scotland is in 1258 when Lawrence and Robert Grant held lands in Nairnshire and Inverness on the Moray Firth. The Grant lands for hundreds of years have stretched for some thirty miles from the hill called Craigellachie at Aviemore along Strath Spey to the village of Craigellachie near where the Spey flows into the Moray Firth — a truly beautiful stretch of country. Craigellachie means ''Hill of Alarm'', for from the top there is a clear view along the river

Spey (the swiftest in the British Isles). There is also a view towards the Cairngorms where approaching enemies could be forestalled as they came through the passes. The war cry of the Grants is ''Stand Fast, Craigellachie!'' The clan has a red feasting tartan, and they wear a hunting tartan similar to the Black Watch Regiment. The clan emblem is the pine tree and the cranberry plant.

Through the female line, i.e., King Robert the Bruce's daughter Marjory, and her son's daughter Margaret, our family are descendants of King Robert the Bruce (d. 1329) and Robert II of Scotland. [*Ian Reid allows that most Scots like to be linked with Robert the Bruce, however tenuous the threads!*]

Grantown-on-Spey, where the Rev. J.C. Grant was brought up, was a new town, conceived by the two Grant lairds, Sir Ludovic and Sir James Grant, in 1766-68. By the 1800s the population had reached 400. From the earliest days, there was a school for boys and a school for girls, as the Scots set great store by children's education.

Groome's Gazeteer of 1885 describes Grantown-on-Spey as a small town in the Inverallan District of Cromdale Parish, Elginshire, within 3/4 mile of the Spey's left bank.[4]

It stands 700 feet above sea-level. By road, it is 34 miles ESE of Inverness, and 24 SW of Craigellachie Junction. It mainly consists of small neat houses of whitish fine-grained granite, so as to equal or excel nearly all other places of its size in Scotland. The site, too, is a pleasant one, in broad Strathspey, with its hills and mountains; and the views are beautiful, away to the far Cairngorms. Surrounded on all sides by forests of pine and birch stretching away southward and eastward, and joining the forests of Ballindalloch and Rothiemurchus, the whole district around Grantown is of the most salubrious character. In no part of Scotland are there more octogenarians and nonogenarians to be met with.

Castle Grant, the seat of the Countess-Dowager of Seafield, stands 2 1/2 miles NNE of the town. It is in the midst of a demesne of more than a thousand acres in extent, thickly planted

> with pines of various kinds. They were brought from all the pine-bearing regions of the world — from the slopes of the Himalayas of Bengal and the Rocky Mountains of America....
>
> Grantown has numerous banks and hotels. It has a cottage hospital, erected by the Countess-Dowager of Seafield in 1884.... It has curling and cyclist clubs, Freemasons' and Oddfellows' lodges, a public library, a horticultural society, the Strathspey Highland Gathering, and an agricultural society. In the vicinity is a distillery, Glenfiddich and Grant....

One great event in Grantown's history was the visit by Queen Victoria and Prince Albert in 1860. They went by coach and stayed overnight at an inn, the Grant Arms. The dinner was described in the Queen's diary as "very fair, and all very clean — soup, hodge-podge, mutton broth with vegetables, fowl with white sauce, good roast lamb, very good potatoes, ending with a good tart of cranberries. When dinner was over, a ringleted woman removed the cloth, and placed the bottle of wine (our own which we had brought) on the table with glasses, which was the old English fashion. After dinner I wrote my diary, and Albert played at 'patience'."

The Grant family maintained a summer home in Grantown until recently. Dr. Grant and his wife Catriona went there often from Canada for summer vacations.

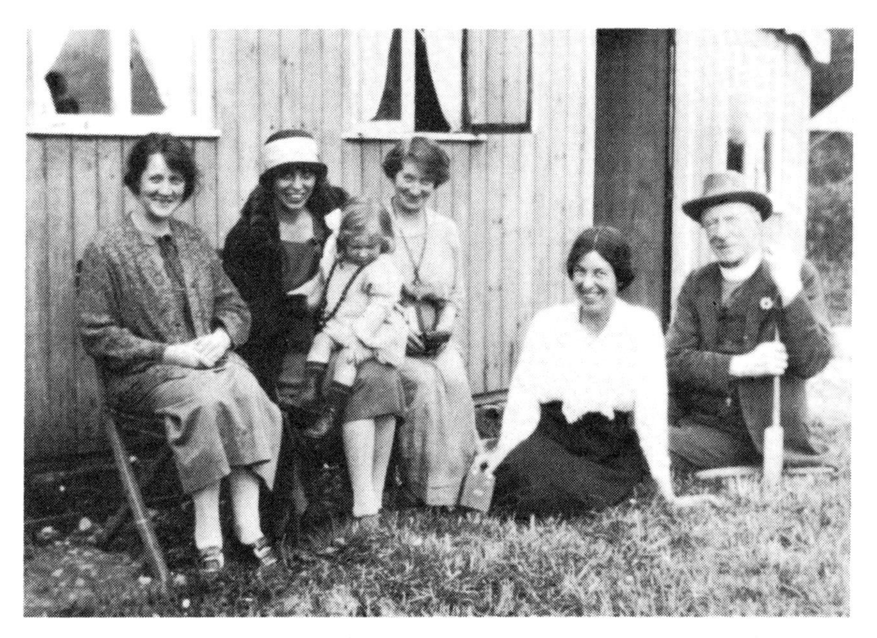

Family taken at the cottage, Grantown-on-Spey: "Poppy" (?), Ellen (?) with child on lap, "Grizel" (?), unknown, and Rev. John.

— Chapter 3 —

Early Years and University

"I ATTENDED the Royal High School, Edinburgh, until the year 1895," Grant writes, "when our family moved to Nottingham, England, where we lived until 1932. There I attended the Boys' High School till 1902, after which I spent a year at school in Grantown-on-Spey."

When he left Mr. Liddell's Classical IVth at Nottingham he stood eighth in the form. He was a classmate of A.W. Adams who later became Secretary to the Ontario Government. It is believed he left the High School because he was not progressing fast enough. At Grantown-on-Spey he probably stayed with one of his aunts, his mother having died two years earlier. Lavinia (Vinny) was his father's sister who had been a Grantown school teacher and who lived in Grantown until her death in 1911.

Grant did not have a strong speaking voice and he was perfectly aware of this handicap as a lecturer. Some people referred to it as "squeaky". The late William Rider, emeritus professsor of radiology and past chief of oncology at the Princess Margaret Hospital in Toronto, who treated Grant's first sub-glottic cancer by irradiation and in whom Grant confided during his illness, referred to his voice as "quaint". Grant had claimed "he could only speak when he exhaled" and that ''his father had become angry with him because of his poor vocal rendition of the Psalms.''

In Nottingham all the Grant children of each sex attended segregated private schools which were a few minutes away from the Manse on Arboretum Street. This must have been a serious drain on a minister's modest income. John's younger brother, Allan, was an exceptional student to whom success seemed to come without much effort. In contrast to John, who was fond of soccer but who did not shine at sporting events, Allan was also an outstanding athlete.

The children of the Manse were expected to be models of decorum, but the burden of good behaviour was sometimes more than they could bear. One of their diversions was to wrap up cold leftover porridge in parcels of brown paper neatly tied with string. They dropped the parcels in the street when nobody was looking and watched from the windows for the first passerby, unable to contain his curiosity, to open a packet. Later, when Grant came home from medical school for a holiday, he might go for a walk with his sister in the evenings down a local lovers lane. He would enjoy startling couples out of their bliss by waving over their heads a skull or other human bone which he had brought home to study.

As a high school student, Grant's seriousness was matched by his dread of appearing conspicuous. His father's insistence on his wearing his kilt to church (in Nottingham) on Sundays so humiliated him in the eyes of other boys that he came to hate it. In the same vein, his extreme modesty made it seem unimportant for him, in later life, to collect his military awards from Buckingham Palace; Mrs. Grant did it for him later.

When his sister, struggling with her homework in the same room, asked John the Latin for some word, she received in reply a lecture on the need to look things up herself. She never doubted this was a matter of principle with her brother, rather than annoyance at an interruption. He was such a perfectionist that when he had difficulty constructing a lucid sentence in English, he would write his message in Latin first and then translate it back into English, satisfied that his grammar would then be impeccable. His fastidiousness was not limited to grammar and syntax. As a lad of fourteen he confided to his mother (shortly before she died) that he preferred to wear navy-coloured clothes so that the least speck of dust on them would warn him that

Session Commencing October 1904, and Terminating March 1905.

No.	NAME		Entry No. of Class Ticket	NATIVE PLACE	PRESENT ADDRESS	Mat. No.	Year of Study	Class Marks	L.	P.	D.	H.	A.	Th.	Ab.	L.
133	Grant	Colin	12	Kirkcaldy	Albert Rd, Richmond	994	2nd			P			X		X	
134	Grant	D. M.	93	Wick	1 Lord Russell Place	498	2nd	2C		P			X	X		X
135	Grant	J. C. B.	102	Scotland	27 Lauriston Place	945	2nd	m 89		P		Xvc	Xvc	2nd MacKenzie Bursary		
136	Grant	J. M.	233	Scotland	24 Spottiswoode St.	619	5th			P			X			

Summer Session Commencing 1st May 1905, and Terminating 19th July 1905.

No.	NAME.		Entry No. of Class Ticket.	NATIVE PLACE.	PRESENT ADDRESS.	Mat. No.	Year of Study.	Cl. Ma.	L.
92	Grant	D. M.	101	Wick	1 Lord Russell Place	498	2nd	–	
93	Grant	J. C. B.	103	Nottingham	37 Lauriston Place	945	2nd	1st	
94	Grant	W. B.	30	Sydney, N.S.W.	7 Polwarth Crest.	353	2nd	1st	
95	Grant	William	256	Ayrshire		2695	4th	–	
96	Guthrie	J. E.	15	Christchurch N.Z.	14 Northumberland St.	2658	1st	–	

Session Commencing October 1905, and Terminating March 1906.

No.	NAME.		Entry No. of Class Ticket.	NATIVE PLACE.	PRESENT ADDRESS.	Mat. No.	Year of Study.	Class Mark.	L.	P.	D.	H.	A.	Th.
162	Grant	D. M.	87	Wick	1 Lord Russell Place	720	3rd	50		P	D			
163	Grant	J. C. B.	180	Scotland	37 Lauriston Pl.	1984	3rd	m 94		P	D		Prosector	
164	Grant	W. B.	21	Sydney N.S.W.	7 Polwarth Crest	561	3rd	84		P			/	
165	Grant	Wm C. M.	53	Edinburgh	7 Alvanley Terr.	1452	1st	20	L					
166	Gray	James	110	Girvan	90 Marchmont Rd.	1978	1st	34	L					

Session 19

HEAD AND NECK.

DATE.			NAME.	ADDRESS.	S.	D.
Dec	13	1	J. L. Wilson	38 Montrose Terr.	4	6
"	"	1	R. H. Jamieson	Elmcairn, Bonnyrigg.	4	6
		1	Fred. Dillon	27 E. Preston Street.	4	6
		1	J. C. B. Grant	37 Lauriston Place.	4	6
"	22	1	G. H. Lowe	47 Leamington Terrace.	4	6
		1	J. D. Ingram	do " "	4	6

Student record, Edinburgh: October 1904—March 1906.

a: It was evidently his work at the head (H) and abdomen (A) which earned him the 2nd MacKenzie Bursary.

b: First class honours (?) with his namesake from Australia.

c: Mark of 94 secured the prosector position. Australian rival close behind.

d: Record of payment (4s/6d) for loan of head and neck specimen.

they needed to be cleaned.

As a medical student too poor even to equip himself with the minimum clothing and boots to play his beloved soccer, Grant discovered his father had been unable to continue to pay Allan's school fees. Somehow John found the necessary money and Allan was able to finish high school. Allan, who understandably idolized his brother, was headed for a medical degree at the time he falsified his age from seventeen to enlist as a combatant in World War I.

In Professor Cunningham's anatomy department, Grant consistently obtained extremely high marks in his class examinations, and was listed in the October 1904 session as having been awarded a Mackenzie Bursary for the second time; this award is still offered for the best student in practical anatomy. The next year he was rewarded by being appointed a prosector in the dissecting room. His excellence in anatomy and his fondness for it ideally suited him for the job. It was an unpaid privilege given to a senior student who had completed the practical part of the course. It involved helping the more junior students to identify structures they were struggling to display, and to execute dissections for mounting as specimens in the teaching museum. Evidently anatomy was his strong suit.

Dr. Grant writes : "I started the study of Medicine at the University of Edinburgh in the year 1903 and graduated MB, ChB in 1908. In our graduating class of 121 students, 8 obtained first class honours and 14 second class honours. I was one of the 14 and one of six entitled to compete for the Allan Fellowship in Clinical Medicine and Clinical Surgery; I competed but without benefit.... In my undergraduate years, I received in Professor Cunningham's class the junior medal in Practical Anatomy, the senior medal in Practical Anatomy, and a Mackenzie Bursary for dissecting."

These achievements were not won without financial cost. In 1905 he signed for a cadaver specimen of the head and neck — the bane of medical students in its anatomical complexity — and had to part with the fee of four shillings and sixpence.

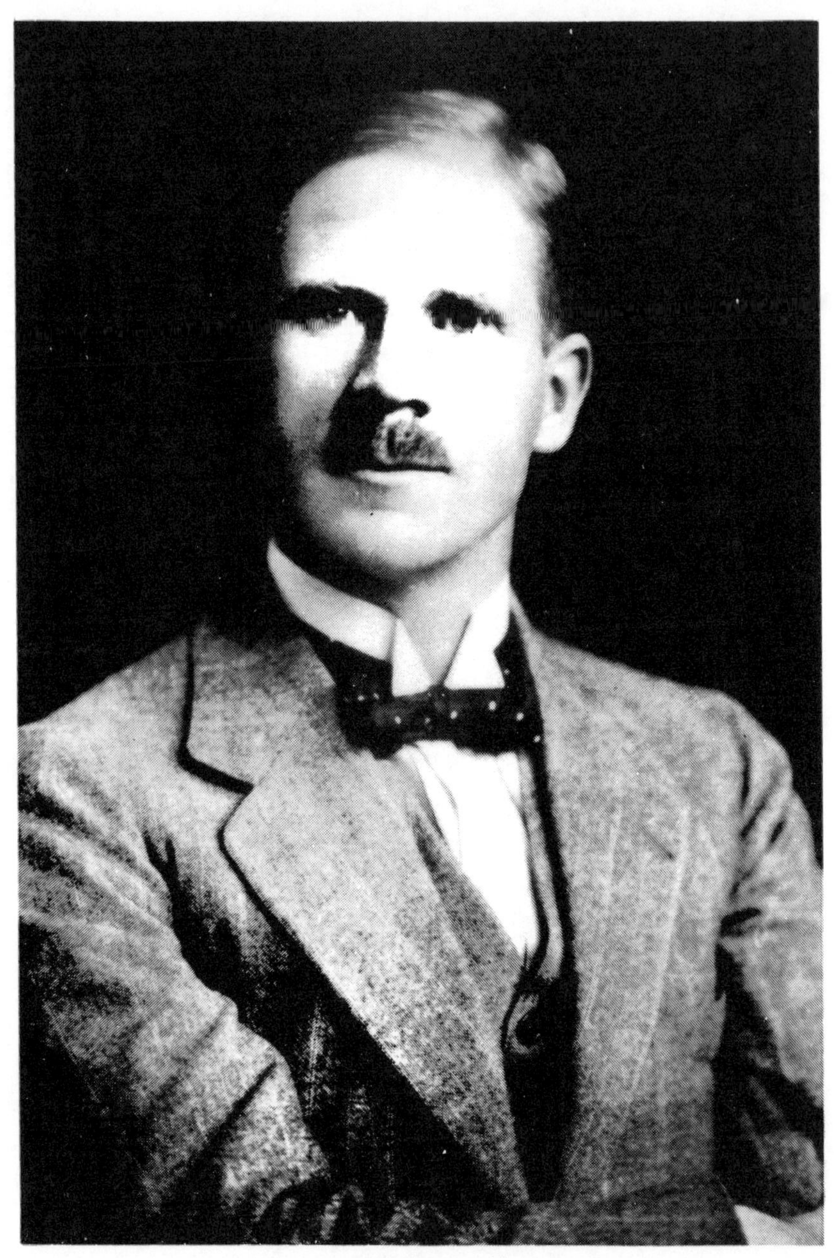

J.C.B. Grant before World War I.

— Chapter 4 —

Doctor in Two World Wars

"DURING vacation periods (Easter, summer and Christmas) in the years 1909 to 1914, I acted as 'locum tenens' in over three dozen private practices and hospitals; my meagre salary of 80 to 120 pounds sterling (i.e., $400 to $600) made it necessary that I should do so." His own account continues:

> War was declared by Great Britain on Germany on the fourth of August 1914. On the next morning I wrote to the War Office applying for a commission in the RAMC, and this I did not receive until the second of November 1914. I was posted to a regiment of the Rifle Brigade, stationed on the Island of Sheppey.
>
> In February 1915, as medical officer I helped to erect the first hospital, 18th General Hospital near Le Touquet, Paris Plage.
>
> In July 1915, I became medical officer to the 1st Battalion, Grenadier Guards.
>
> On 9 September 1917, I asked to be transferred to the 9th Division, for the reason that my remaining brother was adjutant to a Battalion in that Division. I was posted to the 8th

Battalion, Black Watch (Royal Highlanders).

Grant does not make it clear for whose benefit he wrote so sparingly of his life. There is no mention in the *curriculum vitae* that a younger brother, Donald, had been killed at Arras in April of the same year, 1917, although some time later and in another context his niece Alison recorded that Donald had been ''blown to bits at Arras''. His body was never recovered. Nor does he mention his brother Ludovic (Louis) at home in Nottingham, who was unfit for military service. Grant's reluctance to mention all the family members in his *curriculum vitae* is reminiscent of similar omissions in his father's memoirs.

> On the sixth of September 1918, I was transferred to the 58th Casualty Clearing Station to do Ear, Nose and Throat work.
>
> On the seventeenth of October 1918, I was transferred to No. 10 Stationary Hospital to continue that work.
>
> On 11th November 1918 came the Armistice.
>
> ''Military Awards''
>
> I was mentioned in Despatches in September 1916, received a Military Cross (immediate award) in September 1917, and a bar to the Military Cross (immediate award) on August 19th, 1918 (2nd army). In April 1919, I was demobilised and returned to Anatomy and Newcastle-on-Tyne.

The exact details of the deed of valour mentioned in despatches has not been recorded, but the ''mention'' appeared in the *London Gazette* on 4 January 1917, signed by General Sir Douglas Haig, GCB, Commander of the British Armies in France, and dated 13 November 1916. Haig had taken over command from General French who had resigned a few months earlier.

The action must have taken place during the last stages of the Battle of the Somme which had been going on for four months. The British were positioned at the north end of the line, the French, fighting brilliantly, on their right flank. The Allies had been advancing slowly until bad weather, ''King Mud'' and thick forest, combined with enemy action, effectively brought them to a standstill a few miles south of Bapaume.

In the following spring and summer the Allies captured Arras and Vimy Ridge in their slow advance and reached the River Aisne to the south. The next objectives in the Ypres salient were Boisinghe in the north (British Fifth Army) and Armentières on the River Lys seven miles to the south (British Second Army).

At Boisinghe, during the third battle of Ypres in September 1917, the Grenadier Guards endured heavy casualties from shelling. The surviving stretcher-bearers were hard pressed. Grant, as medical officer to the 8th Battalion, rather than waiting for the wounded to be brought to the Advanced Dressing Station, went forward into no-man's-land, "dressed the cases himself on the spot, sending them back as opportunity arose and stretchers turned up. By this gallant act of devotion he undoubtedly expedited the evacuation of the wounded from the shelled area."

For this "conspicuous gallantry and devotion to duty during attack", the Military Cross (immediate award) was given to T./Capt. John Charles Boileau Grant, MB, RAMC.

The second time Grant received an immediate award of the Military Cross was at Meteren on 19 April 1918. It was during Ludendorff's last great German offensive which reached as far south as Château Thierry and Rheims and lasted all through the summer and autumn until Germany capitulated.

On this occasion Grant earned the bar to the Military Cross "for conspicuous gallantry and devotion to duty. He attended to wounded men lying in the open under heavy fire, and subsequently for three days and nights, with little rest, he was constantly out with stretcher-bearers searching for and removing the wounded. He was undoubtedly the means of saving many lives, and his fine example was of the greatest value at a very trying time." The understatement at the end of the last sentence of the official citation would have appealed to Grant.

Allan, for whom Grant had gone to such fraternal lengths to finance his education, was referred to by Grant as his "remaining brother", to the exclusion of Ludovic, after Donald had been killed at Arras. Allan was serving with a Black Watch regiment in the 9th division when Grant's request for a transfer to join him was approved.

Grant did not reveal his views on the morality or immorality of war. There is no commentary from his lips or pen on the justification of imperialistic conflict waged, as all wars are, when one country treads

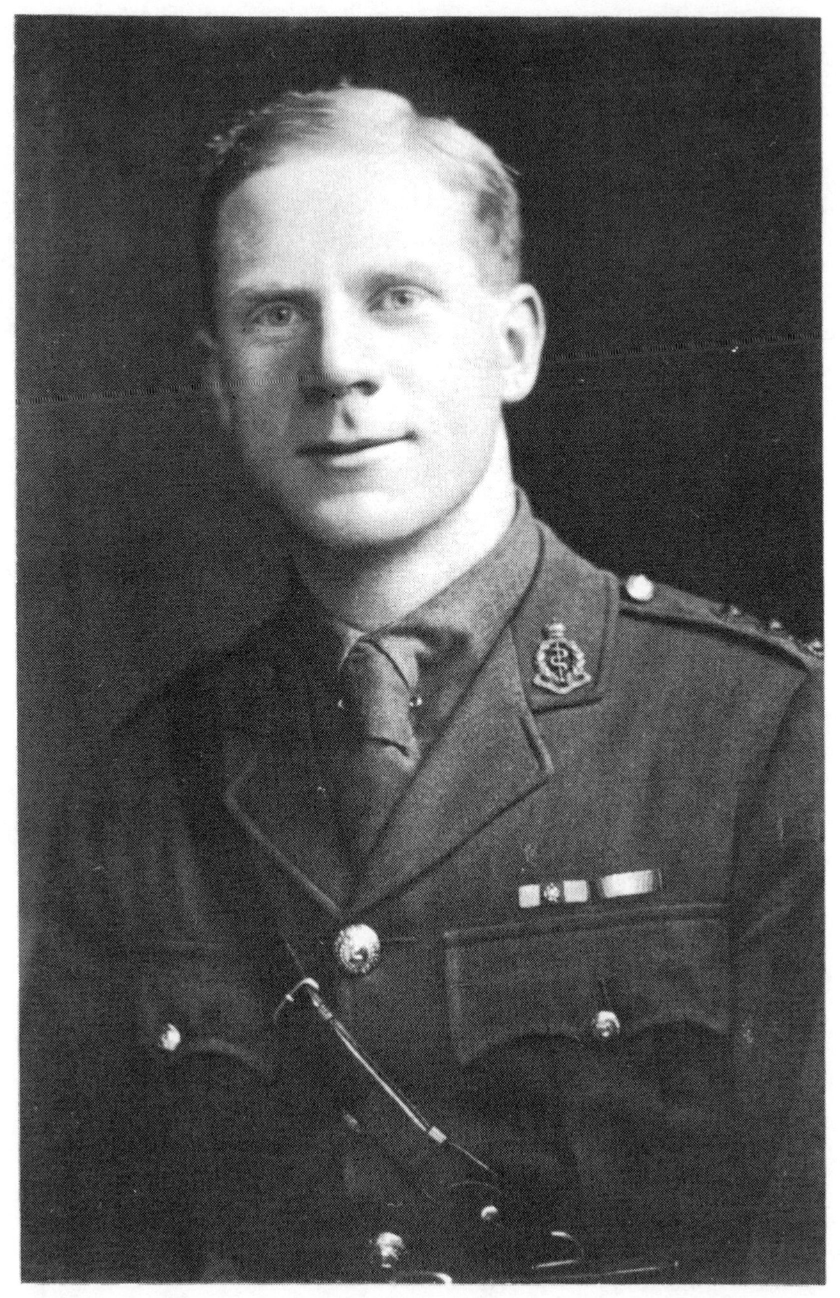

Captain J.C.Boileau Grant, MC and Bar, 1918 or 1919. Note the RAMC badge on the lapel, the MC and Bar ribbon and the General Service ribbon. He does not bother to put up the oak leaf cluster of the Mention in Despatches.

on a neighbour's toes. When Britain declared war in 1914, Canada automatically followed. Canadian contingents serving on the Western Front were all made up of volunteers, half of whom, like Grant, were British born. Imperial fervour was at its height and the correctness of rallying to the flag in response to an enemy's challenge was not questioned. "My country, right or wrong," was the jingoism of the hour.

Canada's sacrifices on the battlefield in World War I forced the British Government to surrender its last vestige of political authority over Canada. Henceforth Canada would not automatically follow Britain in matters of imperial policy, particularly when it came to war. In 1939 the Canadian Government under MacKenzie King exercised its statutory right to autonomy by delaying its own declaration of war against Germany by seven days.

Stephen Leacock, discussing the motives of Canadian volunteers in World War II, wrote: "If you were to ask any Canadian, 'Do you have to go to war if England does?' he'd answer at once, 'Oh, no'. If you then said, 'Would you go to war if England does?' he'd answer, 'Oh, yes'. And if you'd asked, 'Why?' he would say, reflectively, 'Well, you see, we'd have to.'"[1] Leacock could as well have satirized the national sentiment at the beginning of the First World War.

Grant, by now Professor of Anatomy at the University Toronto, again volunteered immediately in 1939. He was rejected on medical grounds because of an inguinal hernia. After he had had the hernia successfully repaired he returned to the recruiting office only to be rejected again. He was told he was more important as a professor of anatomy than a "garrison medical officer", which was as active a posting as he could expect at his age. He accepted the verdict with good grace and resumed his university duties.

— Chapter 5 —

Siblings and Descendants

THE ELDEST in the family, Ellen or "Nellie", was born on 24 May 1884 and died in 1963. She was only 15 years old when their mother died. Although her father employed a housekeeper for a time, Nellie played an important part in the Manse by bringing up the other seven children. In 1910 she married Dr. Alexander Christie Reid, son of another Manse, from Dundee.

After graduating in medicine from Aberdeen University Dr. Reid had moved to England and at the time of his marriage was in general practice in Nottingham. Soon after this he gave up his practice to specialize in ophthalmology. For nearly thirty years he was honorary surgeon at the Nottingham and Midland Eye Infirmary where he carried out research and wrote on nystagmus among coal miners. They had five children, and Nellie spent nearly all her life as a mother and housewife in Nottingham. She and her husband were active in the Belgrave Square Presbyterian Church where her father remained the minister until 1932 when he reached seventy-eight. When she was about seventy-four, Nellie lost her memory.

During the 1950s and 1960s, Ian Reid would come home to Nottingham on leave from teaching in Kenya to find Nellie believing him to be her brother John. Meanwhile, her husband Alexander had died in 1950.

They had had five children, four girls and Ian, the only boy. Ian

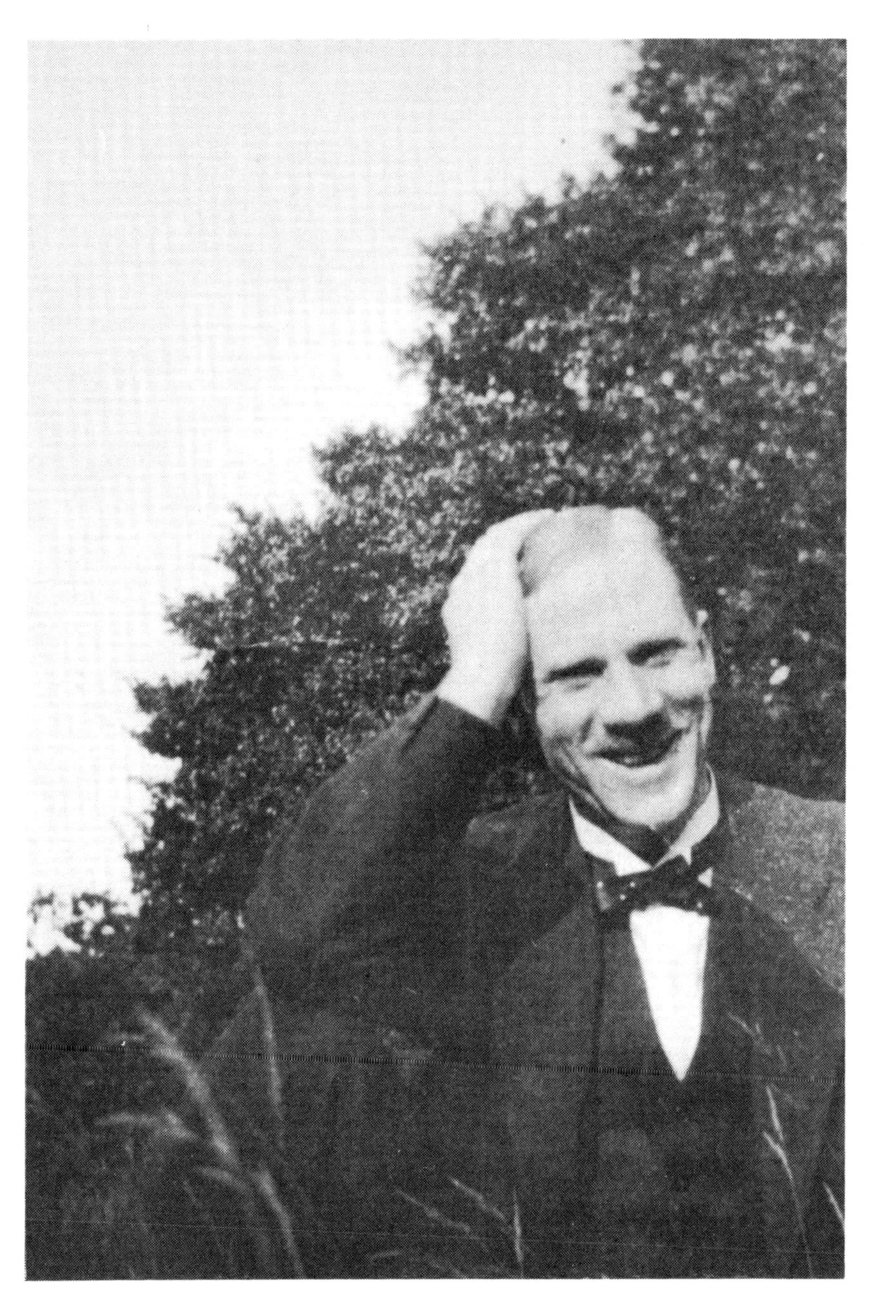

J.C.B. at Golders Green, London, 1924.

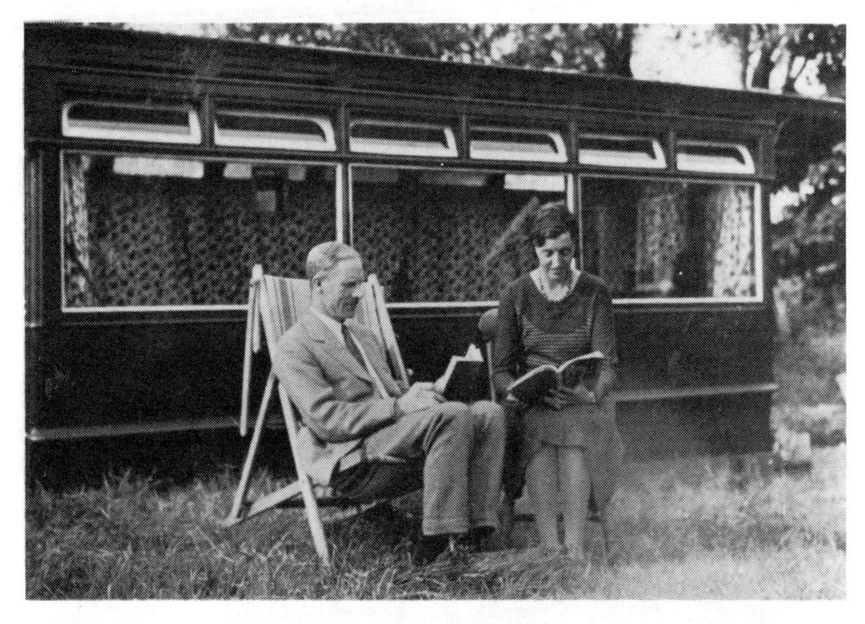

J.C.B. and Catriona outside the summer cottage, Grantown-on-Spey.

reached the rank of major during his six years in World War II in the Black Watch, the senior of the highland regiments and one with early Grant associations. John Grant had been attached to the 8th Battalion in the first war and was still subscribing to the regimental magazine, *The Red Hackle*, up to his death. Ian started his teaching career in 1948 at Nottingham High School where his uncle John had been a student fifty years before. After his marriage to Barbara Herian they moved to Kenya, where he taught for another eleven years, migrating to Canada in 1964. Two children were born to them in Kenya, a son and a daughter.

In 1964 they moved to Ontario where, until 1983, Ian taught classics at Hillfield College, a private day school. Ian's son, Donald, working for the World Wildlife Fund, has studied brown bears and pandas in the Chinese Himalayas. Donald's sister, Anna, graduated in medicine from the University of Ottawa and went into family practice in Vancouver.

Ian recalls J.C.B. Grant:

> I hardly knew my Uncle John in my early years as he had left Britain for Canada before I was born. My memories of him are as an uncle in Canada, with a champion ice-skater wife, who never failed to send a Christmas present to me and my sisters. I remember also the crate of Red Delicious apples from Canada that was delivered to our house every December. Uncle John and Catriona did make at least two trips to Britain in the 1930s, when they spent some time in Nottingham and also stayed at "The Cabin", his father's summer cottage in Grantown-on-Spey. It was not until our arrival in Canada that I really got to know them. By that time, 1964, they had sold their house in Bedford Road, Toronto, and had moved into a beautiful new house at 74 Arjay Crescent, right on the edge of an arm of the Don Valley ravine, north of the city limits, and next door to William Boyd and Enid, Catriona's sister. They entertained us there several times during the summer (they were away in California during the winters), and it was in their garden in June 1973, that I took what was probably the last photo of John, with Catriona, before he died....
>
> John was always a charming host and very interested in

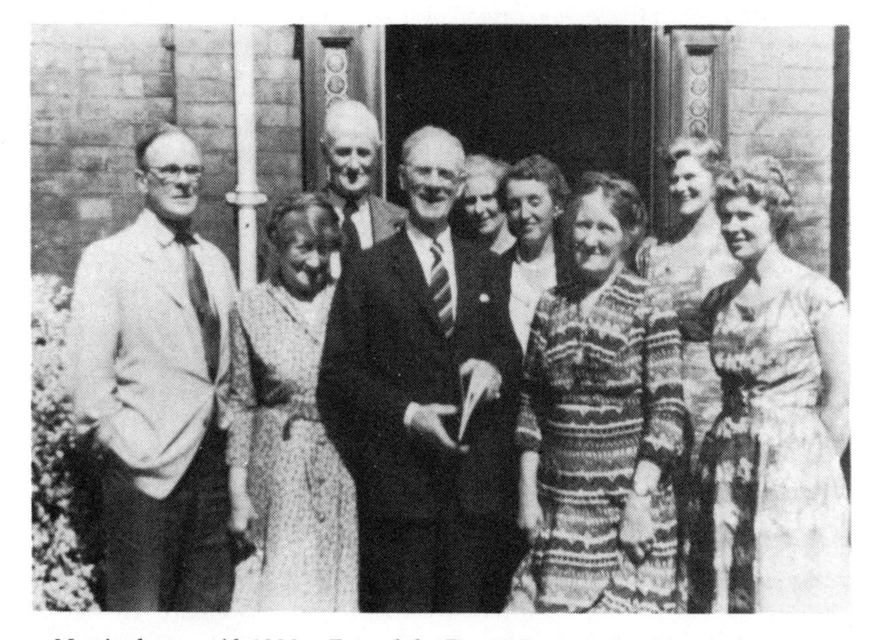

Nottingham, mid-1930s. From left: Dr. A.R. Montgomery, nephew by marriage; Mrs. Mary ("Poppy") Morton née Grant; Col. E.C. De Renzey-Martin, nephew by marriage; J.C.B.; Alison Lofting née Reid, niece; Catriona; Mrs. A. Christie Reid (Ellen or Nellie) née Grant; Mrs.Helen Montgomery née Reid, niece; Mrs. Margaret De Renzey-Martin, née Reid, niece.

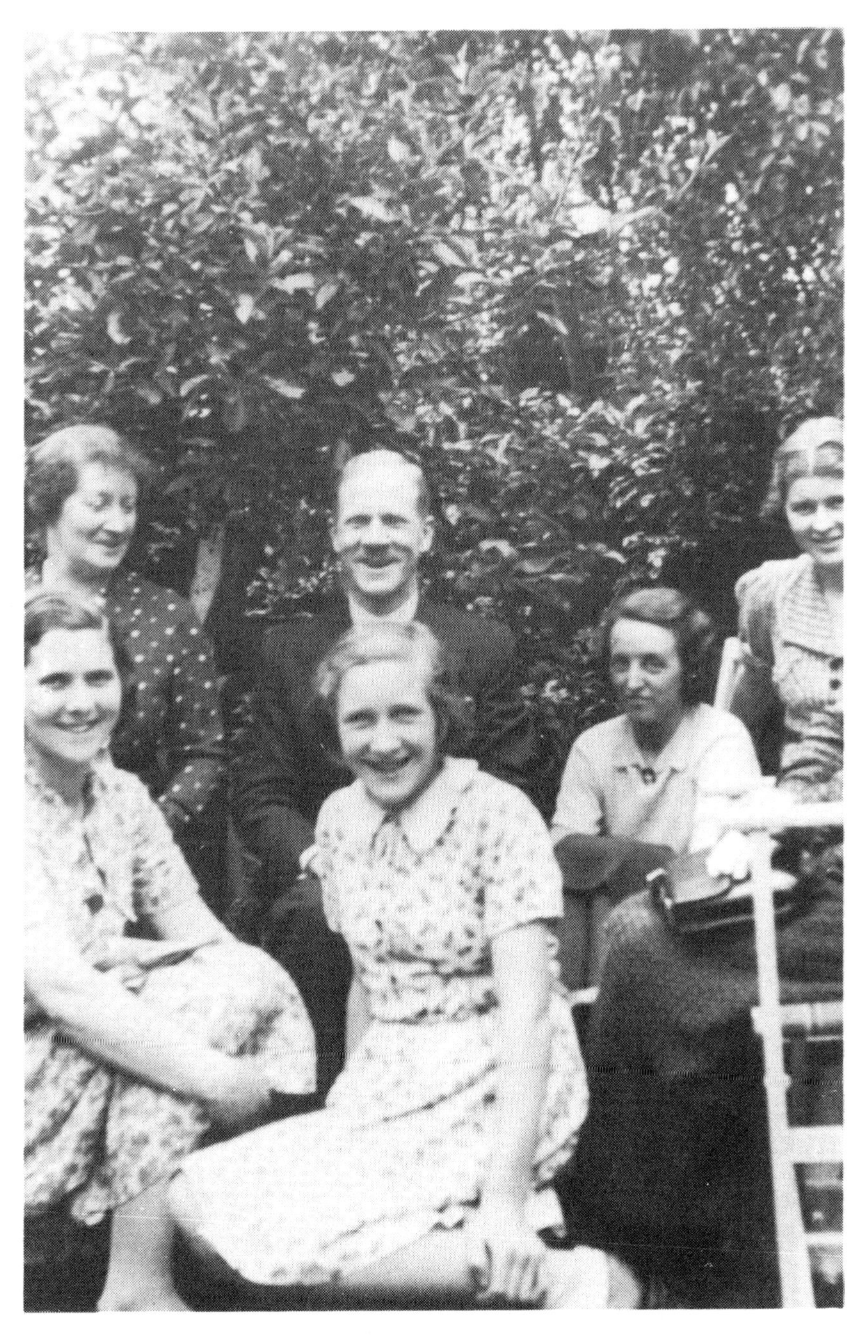

Back row: ''Poppy'' (Morton), J.C.B, Catriona, Margaret (Reid); Front row: Alison (Reid), ''Molly'' (Morton) circa 1936

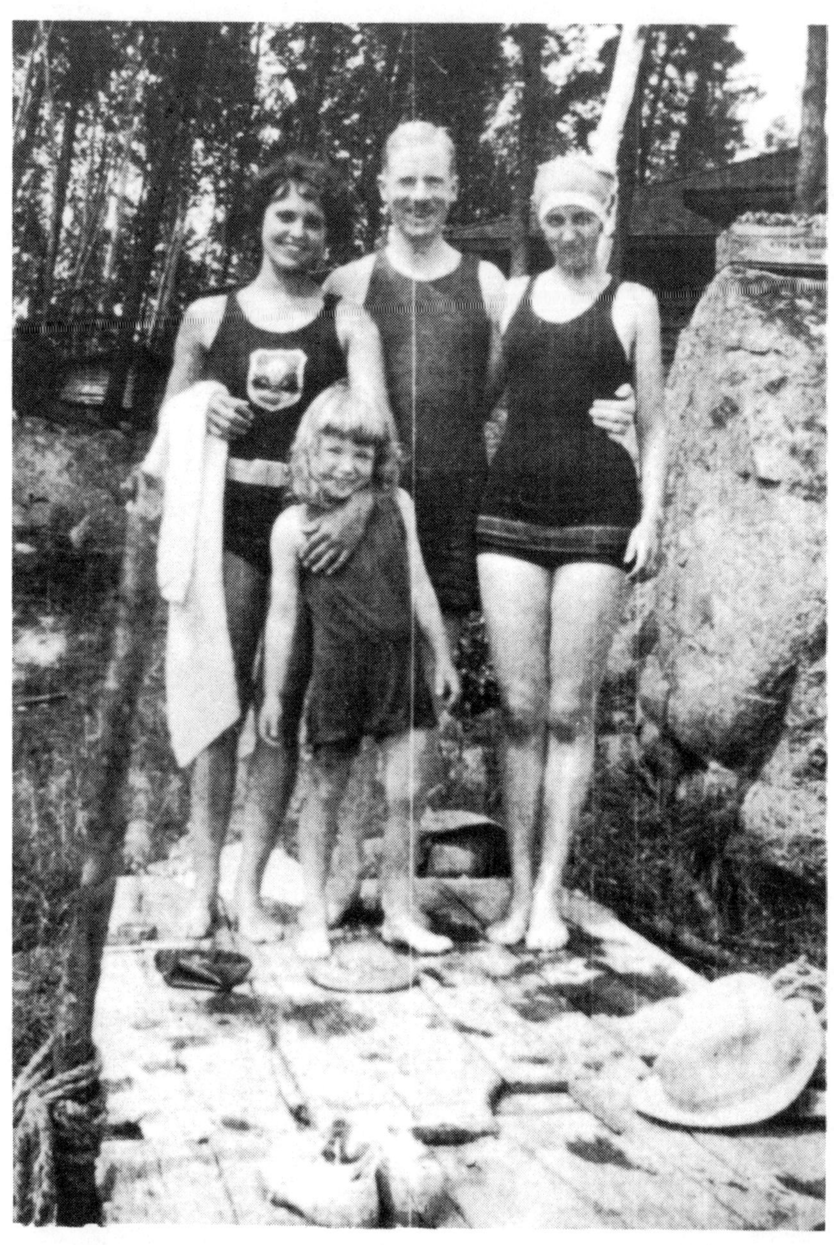

Summer Camp, Lake Winnipeg, circa 1925: Margaret (Christie) Feir, holding daughter Cleone, J.C.B., Catriona. It was here J.C.B. taught Cleone to swim by hanging her from a pole at the end of the dock.

the family and everything we were involved with. They occasionally made the trip to our house in Dundas or to my sister's house in Oakville, but after 1970 they felt they could no longer face the traffic.

I know how greatly Uncle John was respected by doctors in many countries, whether they had studied under him, or met him personally or used his textbooks. I remember a visit to a doctor of East Indian origin in Australia, when my wife and I needed some inoculations. I think I saw Grant's *Atlas of Anatomy* on his bookshelf and remarked that the author was my uncle. He seemed so delighted to know this and was full of praise for the *Atlas*. When we left after our ''jabs'' he said—''That has really made my day, meeting the nephew of Dr. Grant.''

Nellie's only surviving daughter, Alison, Ian's sister, lives in Nottingham:

My reminiscences are mainly of Uncle John's and Aunt Catriona's occasional summer visits when they stayed with us, or at the Manse in Nottingham. I remember him as a courteous, friendly, quietly spoken uncle willing to listen to my schoolgirl prattle. The war years brought these visits to a temporary stop. His last visit to Nottingham was (I think) in the 1960s when my mother was almost too confused to recognize him, which was sad as they were close together as children.

Two trivial incidents I recall. There was a pile of ironing to be done. As my mother was busy with the guests from Canada I thought I would try to help her. Irons in the 1930s were not thermostatically controlled and I singed Uncle John's shirt collar (they were detachable cotton collars in those days). I confessed and expected to be reprimanded but neither Uncle John nor my mother scolded me.

The other remembrance was on a Sunday afternoon at the Manse. Uncle John had been going through some rubbish in a top room and came across a shell from World War I; he felt it was not a safe object to have in the house, so he and I took a tram two and a half miles to Trent Bridge where he threw it in the river. I expected it to blow up the bridge and was ready to run to safety. For all I know it is still lying under Trent Bridge; it was probably as dead as a doornail. The journey home by tram was relaxed and full of laughter.

In 1967 my husband (also John) and I spent three weeks in Canada, the first two nights with John and Catriona. He took us to see his anatomy museum in Toronto University and to their local sports club. That was the last time I saw him, but, as the self-appointed family scribe, I sent him a copy of the family newsletter five or six times a year and a Scottish calendar at Christmas; he sent John and me a subscription for the *National Geographic Magazine*.

Cleone Stoloff, a niece on Catriona's side, and daughter of Mary (Christie) Feir, who died in 1991, writes:

As far as reminiscences go, it is very difficult to write them down as they are sketchy, ancient, and vague. Uncle John was keen on exercise and kept fit and lean. One time when my husband was in Los Angeles on business, Uncle John being there, Catriona and John invited him to Westwood Village for dinner. My husband Alfred was late, having had a drink or two with his colleagues after work; John and Catriona had had a couple more waiting for him so their first meeting of one another got off to a jolly start with more drinks and an exchange of exercise demonstrations on the floor before dinner!

During a much earlier period, about 1925, when my mother went abroad and I was their guest in Winnipeg in summer — I was a little girl — Uncle John taught me to swim. He also built me an exercise bar out of birch poles and taught me how to use it. Uncle John was particular about his eating habits — avoided restaurants, shared a boiled egg with Catriona at breakfast! — and often spoke to me about eating too fast.

He collected oriental rugs (or was it Catriona?). He had various pieces of brass which I am told his father got in the Orient.

At some point John and Catriona took a sabbatical abroad — Austria, Germany? He wrote gracious thank you letters in a beautiful script. He had a great wit and loved to laugh; he

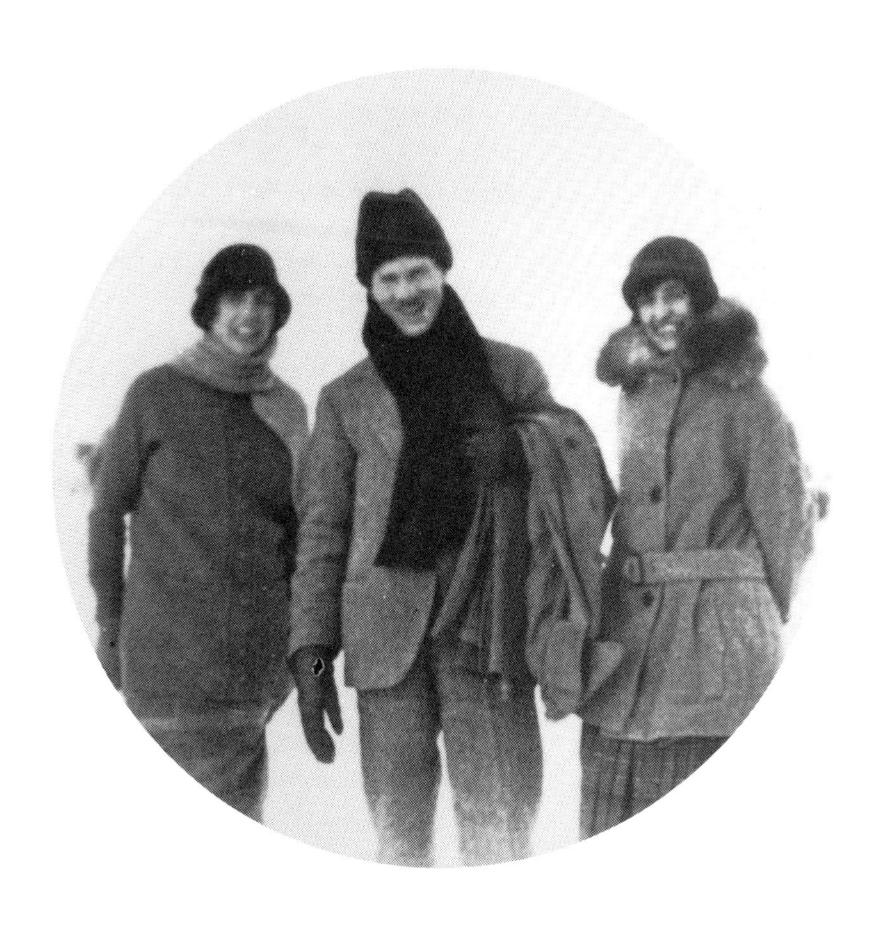

Mary (Christie) Feir, J.C.B., Catriona at Winnipeg.

adored Catriona as is obvious from the photos. He must have been a practical joker — one time in the twenties my father and I were walking behind John and Catriona on a railway track while out picking blueberries at the lake. John and Catriona were ahead and had gone round a bend when a train passed through. When my father and I got round the bend, Catriona was lying on the track as if she were dead — staged by John. My father was not amused!

I also recall that in the Grant household there was a great respect for his illustrators, whose skills were essential to his books. Whether I remember them speaking of Mrs. Dorothy Chubb (first two editions of the *Atlas*) or Miss Nancy Joy (next three) I do not know. Dorothy Foster Chubb's address is listed in connection with Catriona's will in Toronto.

Because so much of John's time was spent on his books Catriona took refuge in fancy ice-skating and became very proficient and skated in a number of ice shows at clubs in Toronto.

A page of Catriona's will, dated 2 July 1980, "undoubtedly reflects John's wishes," Cleone asserts:

> ...consumable stores and all automobile and accessories thereto then owned by me, I bequeath to my sister, Enid G. Boyd, if she survives me, it being my wish that my sister disposes of them as she may think fit.
>
> (b) To transfer, assign and set over to the Ontario Cancer Institute all my right, title and interest in and to the share of my late husband, Dr. J.C. Boileau Grant in royalties in the medical text known as 'Grant's Atlas of Anatomy', it being my wish that the same be used for research and development and the provision of medical equipment, instrument aids and devices necessary or desirable in the work of The Princess Margaret Hospital for the treatment of cancer and the determination of its causes....

The other three Christie sisters are no longer alive. Margaret, who married Col. "Bertie" De Renzey Martin, died in 1974; Helen, the wife of Dr. Alex Montgomery, in 1985. Sheena, married to Ian Reimers, had lived in Oakville, near Toronto, until 1988 when she died, as had Helen, of cancer of the pancreas, a very unusual coincidence.

Grant was the second of his family's siblings; the next was Mary, always known in the family as "Poppy". Mary was the mildly Bohemian member of the family. Before World War I she left Nottingham for London where for a time she worked for Alfred Harmsworth, later Viscount Northcliffe, the newspaper magnate. She was very interested in literature although her work was purely of an editorial and research nature. Mary and her husband Ninian Morton have two children both of whom are now in the U.S.A. — Joan is a nun at Dighton, Mass. and her younger sister Mary ("Molly") lives not far away in Providence, R.I., where her husband, Dr. Harry Kolsky is a professor of physics at Brown University.

Molly has many anecdotes about her uncles John and Allan.

> When I was nine years old, in 1932, Uncle John and Aunt Catriona stayed with us in London for a few days on their way home from a conference in Belgium. I was thrilled (my mother was horrified) when Uncle John gave me the chewing gum an air hostess had given him to protect his ears during landing. I also received from him a lecture on tooth-cleaning, with a demonstration of how to brush up and down from the gums, not from side to side!
>
> There was another visit several years later, in 1939. My father having died rather suddenly, Uncle John paid a late spring visit to make sure that my mother didn't need help. My father had been a civil servant; on his death my mother received no pension from the government but, instead, a sum equivalent to six months of my father's salary. Uncle John provided an annuity for my mother. Thanks to him and my aunt Dorothy Coates, née Grant, I could take advantage of the scholarship I won to London University in 1940.In 1963 we learned that my mother had terminal cancer. My husband and I had emigrated by then with two of our sons when Harry had received a professional appointment at Brown University. I flew over to see my mother in Eastbourne, where she was in hospital. I was startled to see Uncle John in an Eastbourne

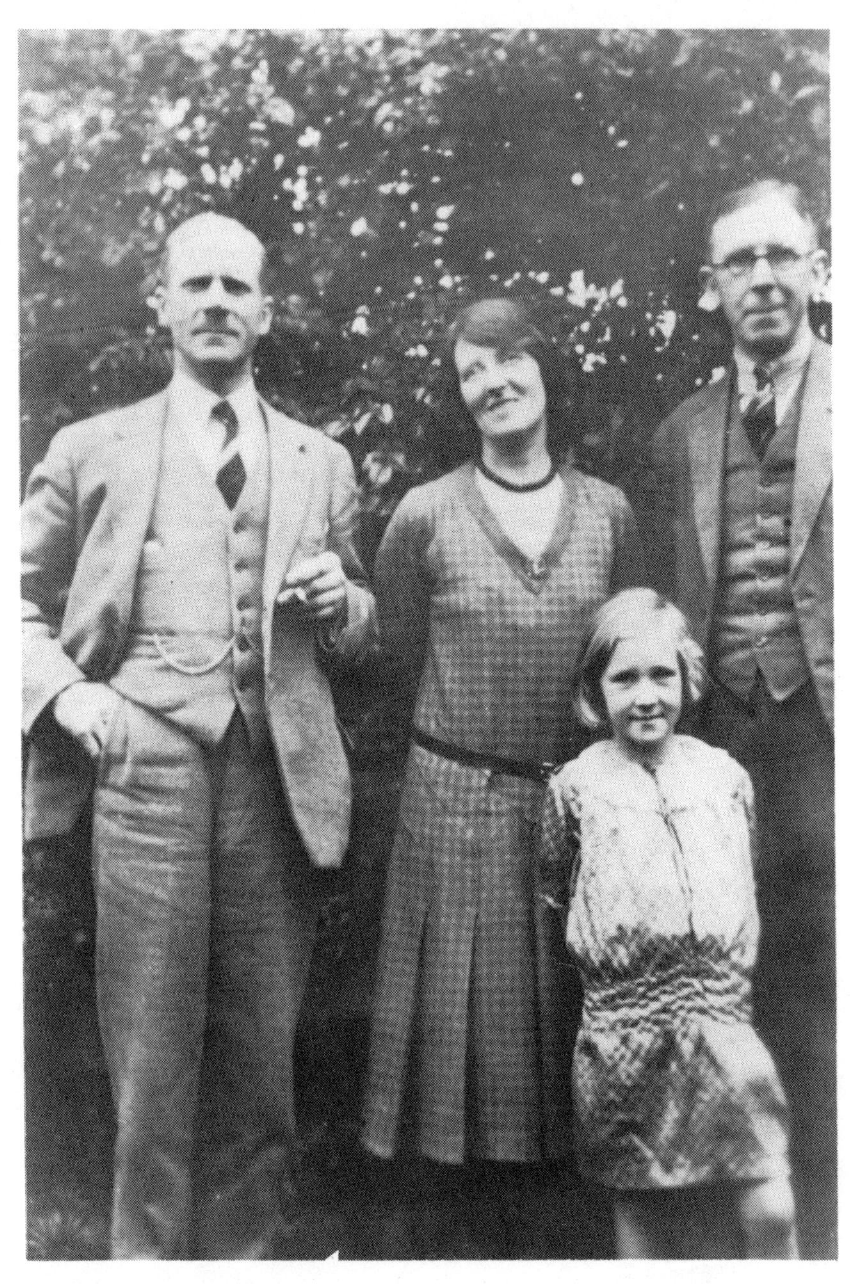

J.C.B., elder sister Nellie Reid, Ninian Morton, and, in front, Mary ("Molly") Grant Morton

street, still walking like a guards officer. He had come to talk to my mother's doctors and to make sure that she had the best available care. He advised me that she should have her gall bladder removed to avoid depression, and I was able to persuade her to do so.

Uncle Allan and his wife ''Bill'' turned up as well, home from a holiday in Venice. They, too, had come to see my mother. For all our sadness and concern, we had what turned out to be quite a jolly luncheon party in Uncle John's hotel—he and Allan were quite devoted to each other and delighted to be together. This gave me some insight into Uncle John's character—self-pity was quite alien to him. It was as much against his principles not to enjoy what he could as it was to wallow in gloom. His distress at his sister's condition was quite separate from his pleasure in reminiscing with his younger brother.

Twice in later summers in the sixties, we drove up to Toronto to see my cousins and Uncle John and Aunt Catriona. I am as shy as he was, and the two of us always found conversation a little difficult. Our middle son, Peter, however, before encountering this somewhat intimidating great-uncle he had never met, had, at the age of fourteen or so, thought of a topic that might suit; he and Uncle John sat there talking nineteen to the dozen about General Gordon and Khartoum.

I remember the pride with which he showed us his little gymnasium in the basement of Arjay Crescent, and the energy with which he attacked the plantains and dandelions which dared to show in his lawn.

I last saw him at home in Arjay Crescent when he already knew he was doomed. Even then, he was most anxious to demonstrate his new garage door-opener, particularly for the amazement of our youngest son, Allan, who cannot have been more than seven or eight. Poor Uncle John could barely swallow at that time and was anxious to conceal this as we had brought a bottle of something or other. He made a gallant pretence of sipping it.

I have just recalled my mother telling me that Uncle John once remarked to her that he never got such good service out of waiters as his fellow guards officers did—he would ask for things rather than demand them.

In my childhood Uncle John was more of a storybook character to me than a real person; I knew my mother hero-worshipped him, but Canada was a long way away. I knew he sent the huge crates of enormous oranges and apples that used to arrive at Christmas. Only after his extraordinary kindness when my parents died did I realize what a very warm person he was for all the shyness and punctiliousness. He and Uncle Allan were boyish when they were together, even in their seventies and eighties.

Of the next brother, Donald Patrick, who was killed at Arras, Ian Reid writes:

Donald has been described to me by those who knew him as a delightful and upright young man. After leaving school he worked in a bank or insurance company in Nottingham. When war broke out in 1914 he enlisted in the Cameron Highlanders. He was killed in action at Arras, and the name 2nd Lieut. Donald Grant is recorded on the great memorial gateway at Menin, at Ypres. It is also on the Edinburgh War Memorial. My son (born 1954) is named after him.

Donald's name also appears beside his mother's on the tombstone in Nottingham.

The next sibling, Elizabeth Dorothy (1891—1945), was a "very gentle and kind-hearted lady":

She ran a very successful one-roomed school from kindergarten to Grade 2 at the Manse, 16 Baker Street, Nottingham. In her late thirties she married Henry Coates, a member of the famous Coats thread family (his father had opened American thread factories in New England and had changed the spelling of his surname by removing the e). They had no children but later adopted Dorothy's orphaned nephew, Robin McGibbon. They lived in Torquay, where her father (Reverend John) and stepmother joined them after her father's retirement in 1932.

The next in line, Ludovic or Louis Nairn Carnethy (1893–1924), was rarely mentioned in family circles unless in hushed tones. He was believed to be mentally handicapped or even to have got into some sort of ''trouble'' with the law. Ludovic's very existence was shrouded in mystery. The next generation of the family hardly ever met him. An occasional glimpse was the only contact with the inhabitant of the top floor of the manse. The children's instinct was that the fewer questions they asked about Ludovic, the happier the household would be. So complete was his isolation that all manner of stories abounded amongst the children. He died when most of his nephews and nieces were children and before the rest of that generation was born. Ludovic's brothers and sisters, including John, evidently did not enlighten their children, which would have dispelled the rumours about him. The few photographs do not look as though he had Down's syndrome nor hydrocephalus, which have been suggested. Even his death did not unlock his secret. The family silence, in keeping with the family's shame, remained absolute.

Whatever the diagnosis might have been there is no doubt that Ludovic — ''Uncle Louis'' — was mentally impaired. One of his nieces remembers the whispered news that Uncle Louis was allowed to sleep in the summer house one summer, but the neighbours had objected because he was ''noisy''. A now ninety-year-old contemporary remembers that Uncle Louis was eager to join the army in World War I like his three brothers. He went regularly to the recruiting office only to be turned away each time. At last a kindly officer presented him with an army cap which he proudly wore, happy that now he was ''in the army''.

Uncle Louis was buried in the same grave as his mother,to be joined later by his sister Grizel and niece Margaret, at the Roack Cemetery, very near to the Baker Street Manse on Forest Road in Nottingham. The cause of death on the certificate was given as ''gangrene and perforated appendix with generalised peritonitis'', and his occupation as ''Gardener—Nursery''. He might well have been a gardener in a mental hospital where, in those days, patients were regularly employed indoors and in the garden and farm, to their own and the asylum's benefit.

The secreting of a ''backward'' child was as common in the early twentieth century as in the 5th century BC when Plato wrote that ''any children that are born defective will be hidden away, in some appropriate manner that must be kept secret. They must be, if the breed of our 'guardians' is to be kept pure."[1] It is doubtful if any age since then in western civilization has shown the tolerance of the later twentieth century towards the mentally handicapped.

Grant and his youngest brother Allan were very fond of each other. Allan turned down a scholarship to Edinburgh University to study medicine and instead, at the age of seventeen, joined the Seaforth Highlanders in World War I, reaching the rank of Major. He served again in World War II and was demobilized with the rank of Colonel. Like his brother John, in World War I he was awarded the Military Cross and bar. The first action took place during the Allies' assault on the Hindenburg line.

Allan's military awards were announced in the *London Gazette*.
MC—26 July 1917
Bar—8 May 1919

MILITARY CROSS
Temp Lt. Allan Roy Stewart Grant
7th Bn., Sea Highrs.

For conspicuous gallantry and devotion to duty. He took command of the company, the remaining three officers being casualties. During the advance he handled his men with the utmost courage and ability under very trying conditions, finally capturing many prisoners.

Place and date) St Laurent Blangy
of deed) 9th April 1917

[Allan's brother, Donald, was killed three days later on the 12th of April in another part of the Western Front.]

BAR TO THE MILITARY CROSS
T/Capt. Allan Roy Stewart Grant, MC
7th Bn., Sea. Highrs.

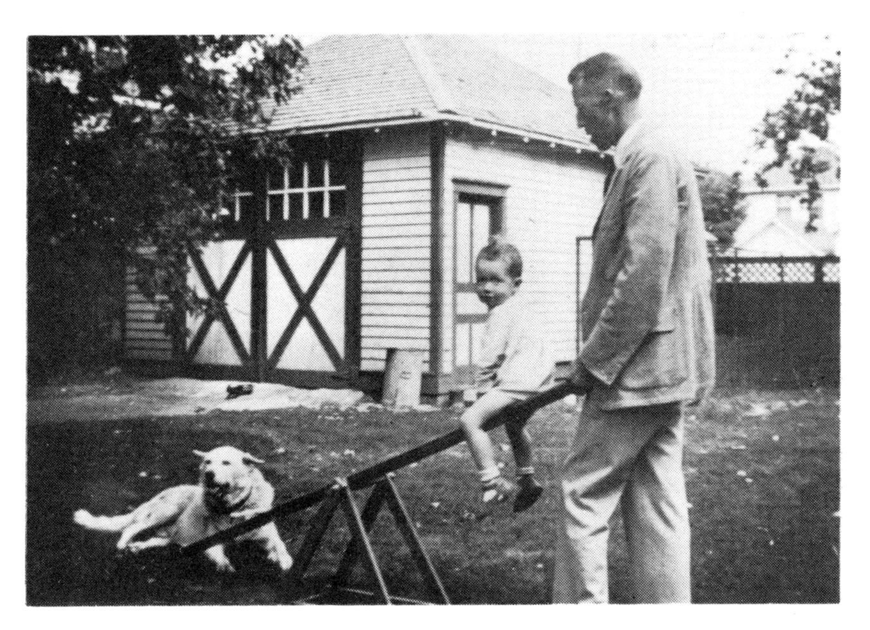

Dr. McGibbon, husband of ''Grizel'', and son Robin at Saskatoon.

> On 20th October, 1918, he led his company with marked skill and gallantry, and when held up by very heavy machine-gun fire near Deerlyck, organized a successful attack on the flank of the enemy position, and then continued the advance to the final objective, which was captured early in the day. Throughout the operations (14th/24th October) he set a very fine example of leadership and disregard of danger.

After World War I, Allan worked for Shell Oil in Liverpool and later in London. His wife Lillian (''Bill'') was a Nottingham girl. They had one daughter, Jean. After Allan's retirement in the early 1960s they moved to Grantown-on-Spey. Here they built a bungalow they called Morar in the field at the back of the old family home, Willowbank. There was already a summer cottage (''The Cabin'', which has since been pulled down) in the same field where the Rev. Grant used to spend the month of August each year. When Lillian was terminally ill with cancer, Jean gave up her job as a social worker to nurse her mother; after her mother's death she looked after Allan, who had developed Alzheimer's disease. Jean continued to live in Morar until her death in June 1988. With Jean's passing, the last link of the Grant family with Grantown-on-Spey was broken.

Grace (Grizel), the baby of the family (1897—1936), ''was a blazing red-head and had a lively personality to match,'' says Ian Reid. She married Dr. Robin Tweedie McGibbon and emigrated with him to Winnipeg, where McGibbon was appointed assistant professor of anatomy under Dr. Grant. Presumably McGibbon, a graduate of Glasgow University, had known about and had even met Grant before the latter had emigrated to Manitoba. The circumstances surrounding the meeting of McGibbon and Grace are not known.

Professor Audrey Kerr, head of the medical library at the University of Manitoba, writes: ''Robert Tweedie McGibbon was appointed here in October 1921 as Assistant Professor of Anatomy. He had his MB, ChB from Glasgow and had worked there for some three years before applying here. He left Manitoba in 1926 to become the first head of anatomy at the University of Saskatchewan. Our archives record neither his birth date nor date of death.''

Archie Christie, a brother of Catriona, tells of the trials of his late brother David in anatomy when he was a medical student at Winnipeg in Grant's time as head of the department. In the year David wrote his final examination in anatomy, McGibbon, as assistant professor, happened to have been given the duty of marking the examination papers. McGibbon failed David, giving him a mark of 49%. (This was the only examination David ever failed.) David wrote a supplemental examination a few months later and passed. Dr. Grant, at the time, would not interfere with the mark that failed David. On the one hand he obviously had sympathy for his brother-in-law, but on the other he was bound to accept his junior professor's judgement. He confided later, however, that he could have re-marked the paper and given David a pass mark, but his probity would not allow him to bend his convictions.

McGibbon left Winnipeg to become the first Professor and Head of Anatomy at the University of Saskatchewan in May 1926. Nine years later, early in the morning of 13 May 1935, his wife found him dead at his desk. He had not returned home the previous evening. He was thirty-seven. The Saskatoon *Star-Phoenix* reported he was preparing a "heavy program of research in brain surgery" with Dr. Lorne McConnell. There was an investigation into his death but no inquest. An autopsy by Dr. Frances McGill indicated death by natural causes. A colleague who had attended the Saskatoon medical school at that time has said that McGibbon died from a massive inhalation of stomach contents.

Grace, having borne one son, Robin, returned with him to Nottingham after her husband's unexpected death. She worked in the radiology department at Nottingham General Hospital. She herself died a year after her husband following an operation for twisted colon.

The last of Grant's immediate siblings was Benoni, "child of my sorrow", who died with his mother at his birth. Grant left no record of his reaction to his mother's death when he was only fourteen. His father, Reverend Grant, married Susan Macy four years later and J.C.B. acquired a half-brother, Charles Baring Travers, who eventually went into general practice at Crawley near London's Gatwick Airport.

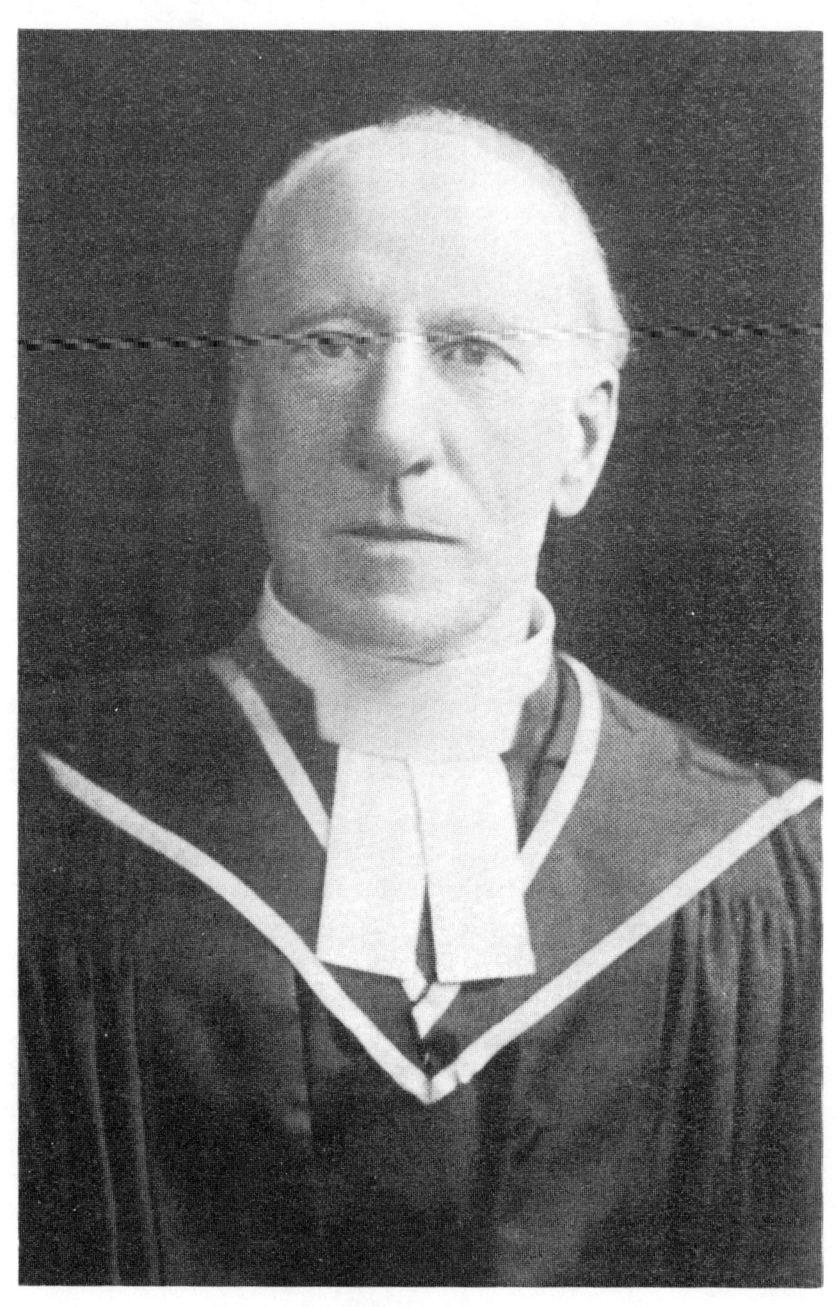

Reverend John Charles Grant.

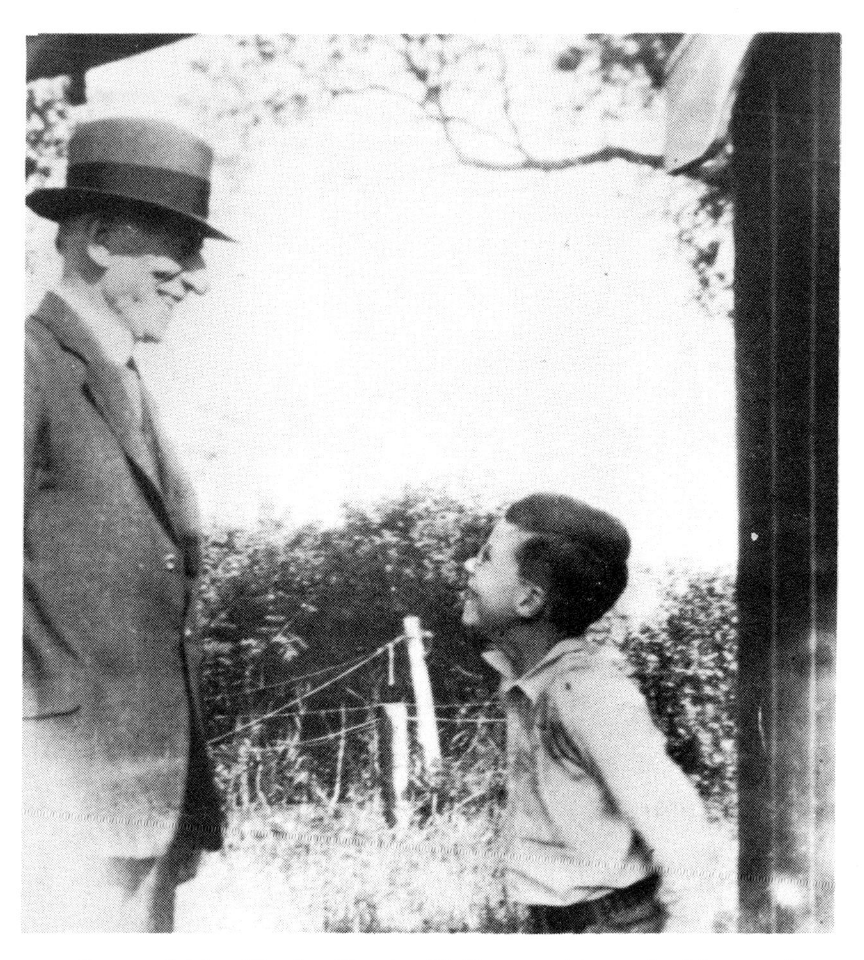

Reverend John Charles Grant with Travers, his son by his second marriage.

— Chapter 6 —

University of Manitoba

"HAVING BEEN invited to apply for the Professorship of Anatomy in the University, at Winnipeg, I did so, received the appointment, and arrived in Winnipeg on 21st October 1919." Grant continues:

> On my first vacation, in June 1920, I first went south to visit the fabulous Mayo Clinic and the University of Minnesota en route; then turning north, as medical officer to the Indian Treaty Party, I went by canoe down the Nelson River to York Factory and Churchill on Hudson Bay.
>
> On finding out that almost no work had been done on the anthropometry (physical anthropology) of the North American Indians of Canada, it seemed obvious that without further delay data on the Indians should be collected before further intermixture with other races took place. So, with the guidance of Diamond Jenness, CC, I made many summer excursions to the Indians living around Lake Winnipeg and in the North West Territories; took various measurements and recorded observations on them. The results have been published by the Department of Mines as Bulletins on Eastern Cree and Saulteaux, Chipewyan, Western Cree, Beaver, Sekani and

Carrier (using Jenness's data)[1],[2]; reports on Stoney Indians and Indians around Lesser Slave Lake have yet to be published. [Apparently they were never published.]

Grant was not the first member of the 1908 University of Edinburgh medical class to go to Winnipeg; Alexander Gibson (1883 - 1956) had preceded him. Gibson had taken an Arts degree at Glasgow University before starting in medicine. In his final year, he had won first class scholarships in the classics and in mathematics, and the first medal in English Literature. He had a remarkable record as a medical student, for he was the first student at Edinburgh University to earn the scholarships available to him in every year. He had gone to Winnipeg in 1913 to be professor of anatomy. When World War I broke out, a year after his arrival, he left to serve in the RAMC in India and Egypt. After war service, he was appointed to the chair of orthopaedic surgery in the University of Manitoba. It was he, with William Boyd and, of course, the Dean who were responsible for the invitation to Grant to join the faculty.

The second member of the Edinburgh medical class of 1908 to go to Winnipeg was William Boyd. Alex Gibson was Boyd's best friend and companion in mountain climbing and his best man at his wedding. It was Gibson who had been mainly responsible for Boyd's invitation early in 1914 to the chair of pathology in Winnipeg. But by the time Boyd got the notice of his appointment he was in France with the RAMC. A year later, he was "requisitioned" by the University of Manitoba and arrived in Winnipeg in 1916.[3]

When Alex Gibson resigned the chair of anatomy and concentrated on orthopaedic surgery, the Dean of Medicine asked him to suggest a successor for the chair of anatomy. Without hesitation he recommended his fellow student from Edinburgh, J.C. Boileau Grant. Grant was by that time an accomplished anatomist whose achievements and ability were already recognized.

Boyd had married Enid Christie in 1917. She was a daughter of the manse; her father, the Rev. David Christie, had taken his education at St. Andrews and Edinburgh before emigrating to Winnipeg. So when Grant arrived in Winnipeg by train in October 1919 Boyd met him at the station and took him home for dinner. Here he met Mrs. Boyd's sister, Catriona, whom, according to Boyd, "he promptly

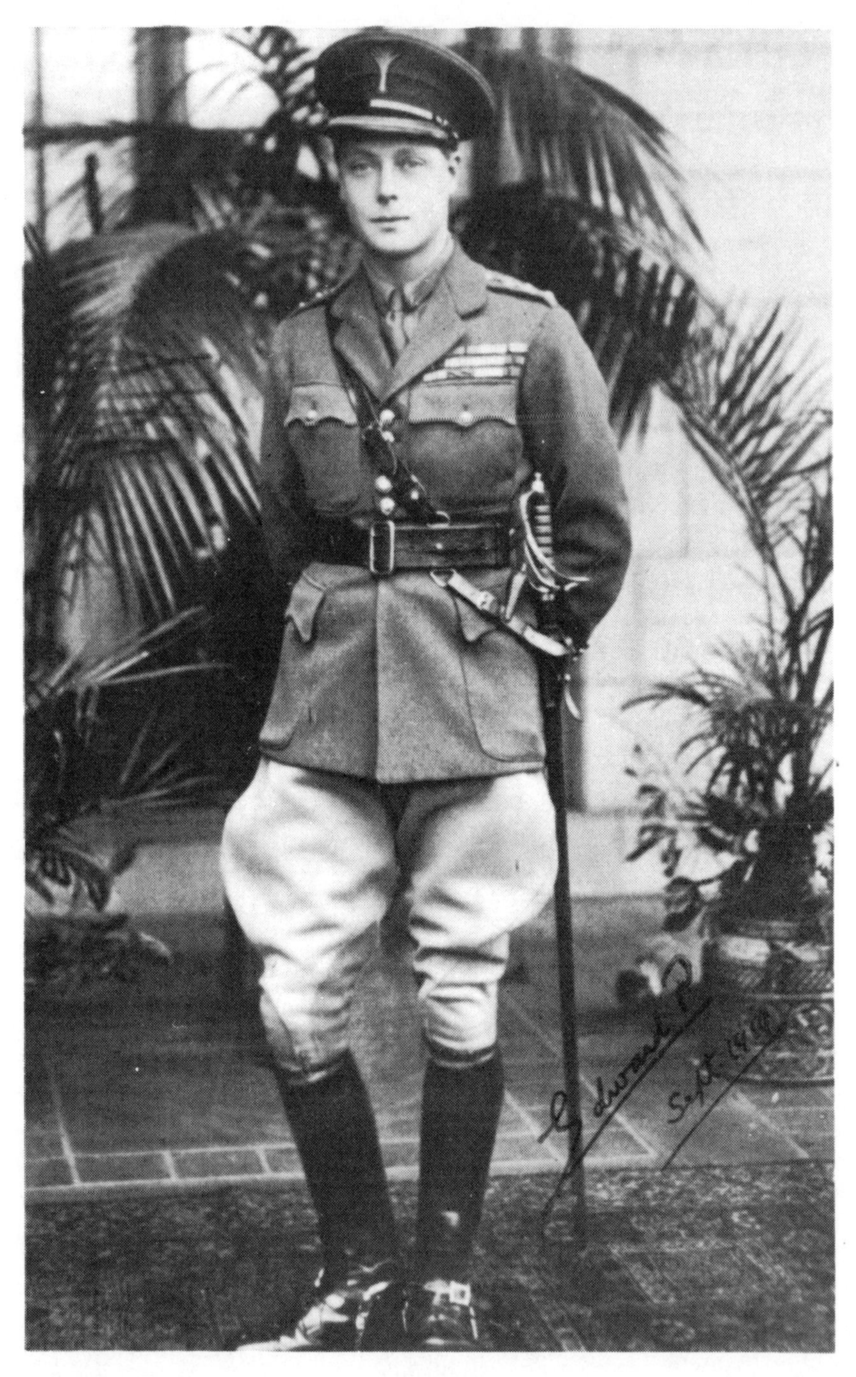

Edward, Prince of Wales, at the time of his first visit to Canada, September 1919, when he arranged the purchase of the "E.P." Ranch near High River, Alberta. The photograph was signed and sent to Catriona. On the back, Catriona has written, "A dance partner, 1919. Catriona and Isobel wearing the same dress on each occasion."

married.'' Well, not quite. They delayed the marriage until 1922.

Apart from their friendship with him, the two new arrivals had good reason to be warmly appreciative of Alex Gibson. ''Any day at noontide,'' Grant wrote, ''you could learn from him all the news in the morning paper, world news, local news, the price of stocks, theatrical news, the bargains of the day as advertised. Nothing seemed to miss his eye.'' He retained that power until the day he suddenly died in his office.

Thus the three medical students from Edinburgh began their university careers in Winnipeg. But for Alex Gibson and the University of Manitoba two of the most famous teachers in the English-speaking world might never have adorned Canadian medicine.

The first visit of the twenty-five-year-old Prince of Wales in September 1919 to Western Canada symbolized the importance of Winnipeg in the rapidly developing country. Grant did not arrive until a month later, but Catriona and her sister Isobel attended at least some of the social functions mounted in Winnipeg in the Prince's honour. The two sisters, according to Catriona, took turns to wear the same dress for the dazzling occasions—or, as Ben, Isobel's son, speculates, they each had a similar dress. In either event, their action was in keeping with their sprightly and rebellious natures.

It was on this tour that the Prince visited Calgary and stayed at George Lane's 6000-acre ranch near High River, Alberta. He marked his admiration for the foothills by planting, amidst much ceremony, a tree brought from the nearby Aldersyde district and by the purchase of 1600 acres, to be known as the E.P. ranch, adjacent to Lane's property. The Prince (later Edward VIII) visited his ranch three more times before his abdication of the throne, and once afterwards, as the Duke of Windsor, with his wife, the former Wallis Simpson. The Duchess was not interested in wide open spaces, however beautiful, and the ranch was sold in 1962 around the time the tree died as symbolically as it had been planted, but with less ceremony. Charlie Clark, the editor of the *High River Times,* wrote in his paper, ''It's a relief that the ranch went to a local man; we know it will be used as a working ranch, to good advantage.''[4]

After Catriona graduated from the University of Manitoba she became a school teacher, a profession she enjoyed. It suited her temperament to impart to her pupils her irrepressible *joie de vivre,* a trait which, even in old age, never flagged. She was an excellent skater and danced on ice with verve, taking her sister Enid as partner rather than not dance at all. Not long after the Grants had moved to Toronto, Catriona, vivacious and gregarious as ever, enquired of medical students where they went for ballroom dancing and learned that the Old Mill was the favourite and affordable spot.

During the summer of 1920 Grant carried out anthropometric studies of numerous Indian tribes in northern Manitoba, navigating the Nelson River by canoe to its outlet at York Factory on Hudson Bay, a trip of about 200 miles. He made several other similar trips in the north during the 1920s. Anyone who has suffered the torture of black flies and mosquitoes of Canada's north country in the summer will appreciate Grant's devotion to research and learning. His findings (to be described in a later chapter) were published in the bulletins of the federal Department of Mines in Ottawa.

J.C.B. Grant and Catriona Christie were married in 1922. The Winnipeg *Tribune* reflected the public enthusiam of the event. Under the headline **POPULAR MIDSUMMER WEDDING** there was a photograph of Catriona in a trailing wedding dress complete with a very long bridal veil and carrying a large bouquet.

> Westminster church, Maryland St., was the setting for a very interesting event Thursday evening, when, at 8 o'clock, Rev. Dr. Christie, assisted by Dr.C.W.Gordon, united in marriage his youngest daughter, Anne Catriona, and Prof. J.C.B. Grant, MD.
>
> The church, which was effectively decorated with palms and ferns, was filled with a large number of interested guests.
>
> At the appointed hour the groom with his groomsman, Dr.Alexander Gibson, took their places, and as the first notes of the Lohengrin wedding march were heard, the bride with her father, who gave his daughter in marriage, moved slowly down the aisle, preceded by her two brothers, James and David Christie. She was attended by her sister, Mrs. James Feir, of Regina, as her matron of honour, and her little niece, Miss Peggy Feir. Her wedding gown was a Parisian model of soft white crepe satin draped with Carrackmacross lace. Her veil of tulle, which formed the long train, was arranged with lace

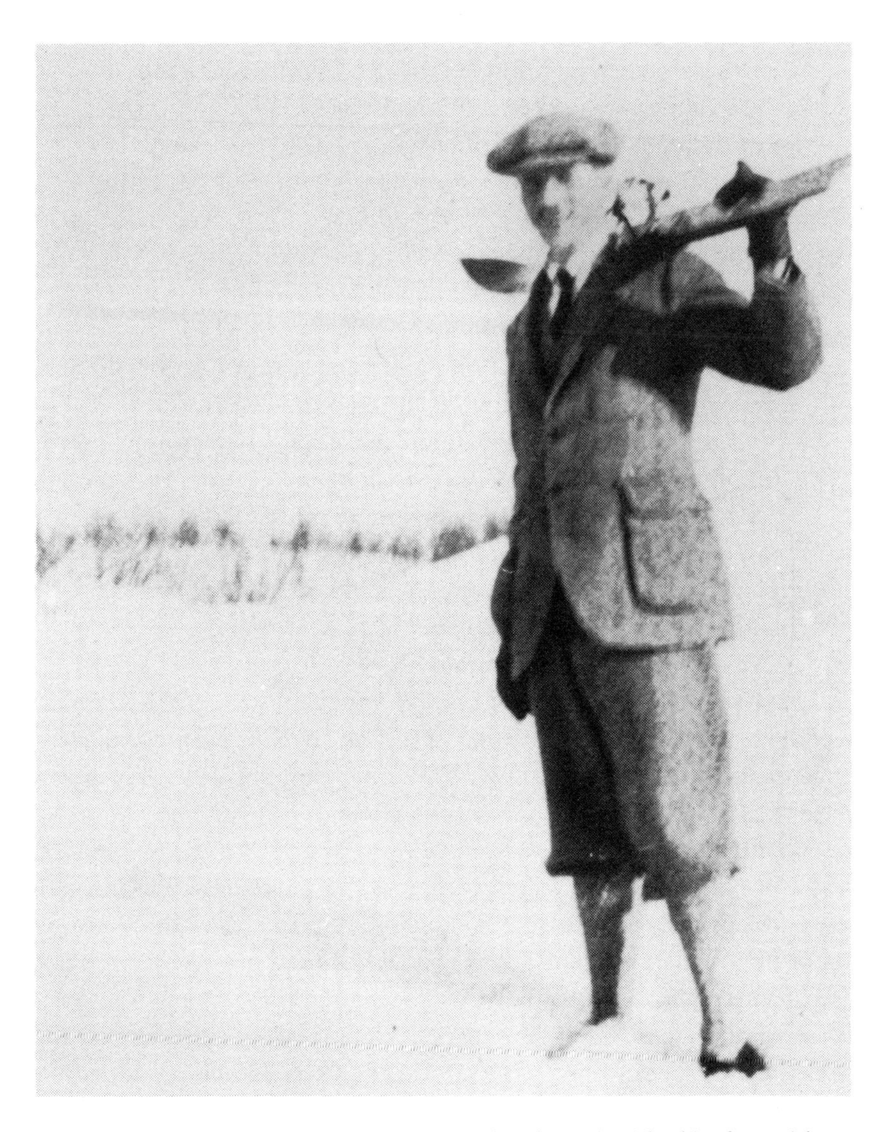

J.C.B., Manitoba. A cheerful pose in "plus fours" with skis, but without poles or boots.

> and orange blossoms. She carried a shower bouquet of pink roses and valley lillies, and wore the groom's gift, a pearl necklace.
>
> The service was preluded by the hymn, ''O God of Bethel'', sung by the choir, which also sang during the signing of the register the wedding hymn, ''O Perfect Love''.
>
> After the ceremony, an informal reception was held at the Manse, Maryland St. The Rev. Dr. and Mrs. Christie presided with the bridal party at the entrance of the drawing room, and in the dining room the bride's table, centred with the wedding cake, was decorated with sweet peas and roses.
>
> Later in the evening Prof. and Mrs. Grant left for an extended honeymoon in Banff, Lake Louise and the coast cities. Mrs. Grant travelled in a smart tailleur of navy blue trimmed with white kid, with a small model hat.
>
> Mrs. Fraser McConnell wore a midnight blue lace dress, with a dark blue picture hat. Mrs. William Boyd's costume was a French model of yellow crepe de chine, with a leghorn hat wreathed with yellow blossoms.

Dr. Grant's father travelled from Nottingham to attend his son's wedding. This was probably his first visit to North America. His expenses and fare were paid by his congregation in Nottingham and recorded as an ''extra'' in the church's books.

Grant's textbook *A Method of Anatomy, Descriptive and Deductive*[5] was started while he was professor and head of anatomy at the University of Manitoba, but was not completed and published until a few years after he had reached Toronto in 1937. In the preface to the first edition he states: ''One method of studying human anatomy is to collect facts and memorize them. This demands a memory which is wax to receive impressions and marble to retain them. The other way consists in studying them with their mutual relationships.'' He continues:

> For example, the markings, lines and ridges, depressions and excrescences, on a bone tell a story as do the scars and irregularities on the earth's surface. Because they are in the main to be interpreted by reference to the soft parts that surround and find attachment to them, the bones are not described together

under the heading ''osteology'' as though they were things apart. The shafts of the bones are considered with the surrounding soft parts; the ends with the joints into which they enter.

Surface Anatomy is not done as an independent subject, but is undertaken as a review of Gross Anatomy, distances being measured, where feasible, in terms of structures. Thus, instead of stating that the posterior tibial artery lies half an inch from the tibial malleolus—which would be a new fact to memorize—it is spoken of as being the breadth of two tendons from the malleolus, the tendons being the tibialis posterior and flexor digitorum muscles—a fact already learned by dissection. Again, by regarding the left renal vein as the vein of the three left paired abdominal glands (adrenal, renal and sex) its length is easily calculated as being the length of the right renal vein, plus the width of the vanished left inferior vena cava, plus the breadth of the aorta, say 1 1/2 + 1 + 1 = 3 1/2 inches; and again, the memory is not strained to remember that the adrenal gland lies at the level of the twelfth thoracic vertebra when the fact can profitably and readily be deduced from a series of related circumstances.

Illustrations to be of value must be simple, accurate, and convey a definite idea. It is for these reasons that they consist entirely of line drawings.

The book is meant to be a working instrument designed to make Anatomy of direct application to the problems of medicine and surgery. The bare, dry, and unrelated facts of Anatomy tend rapidly to disappear into forgetfulness. This is largely because its guiding principles are not grasped so as to capture the imagination. Once they are grasped it will be found that details and relationships will remain within certain and easy recall.

With the same concept of deductive reasoning, Grant read a paper at the 38th annual meeting of the Association of Anatomists held in Montreal in October 1927. It was entitled ''The teaching of anatomy at the University of Manitoba''[6]. It is a fairly long paper and would have taken more than the usual ten or fifteen minutes alloted to a paper

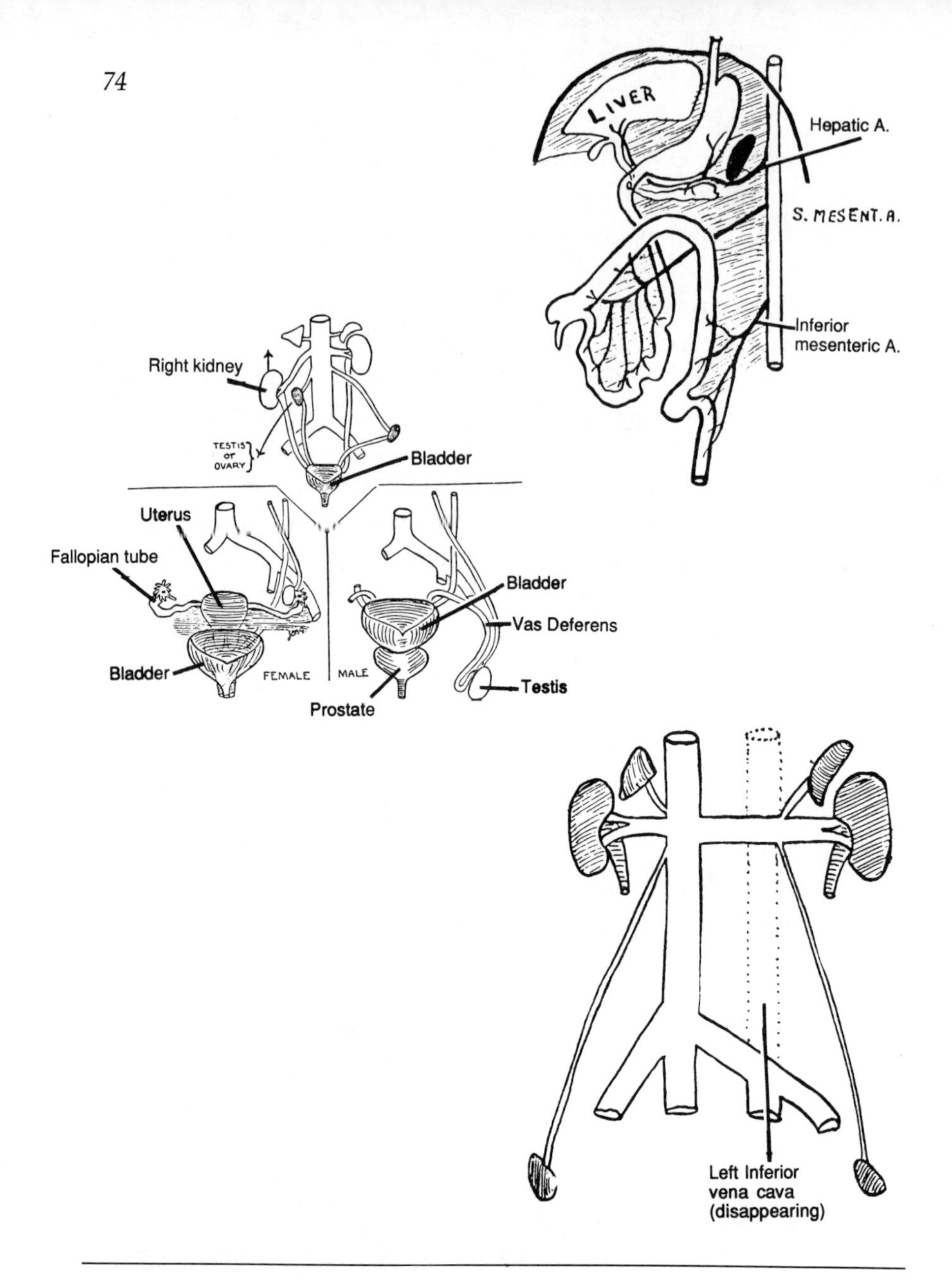

Anatomical relationships. University of Manitoba, 1925.

a: Rotation of gut—initially hanging from dorsal mesentery, then, rotation to the right.

b: The descent of the testes and the ascent of the kidneys; showing the testicular and ovarian ducts in front of the ureters.

c: The assimilation of the left vena cava, and the subsequent venous drainage of the adrenal and testis; the longer left renal vein and the longer left common iliac vein.

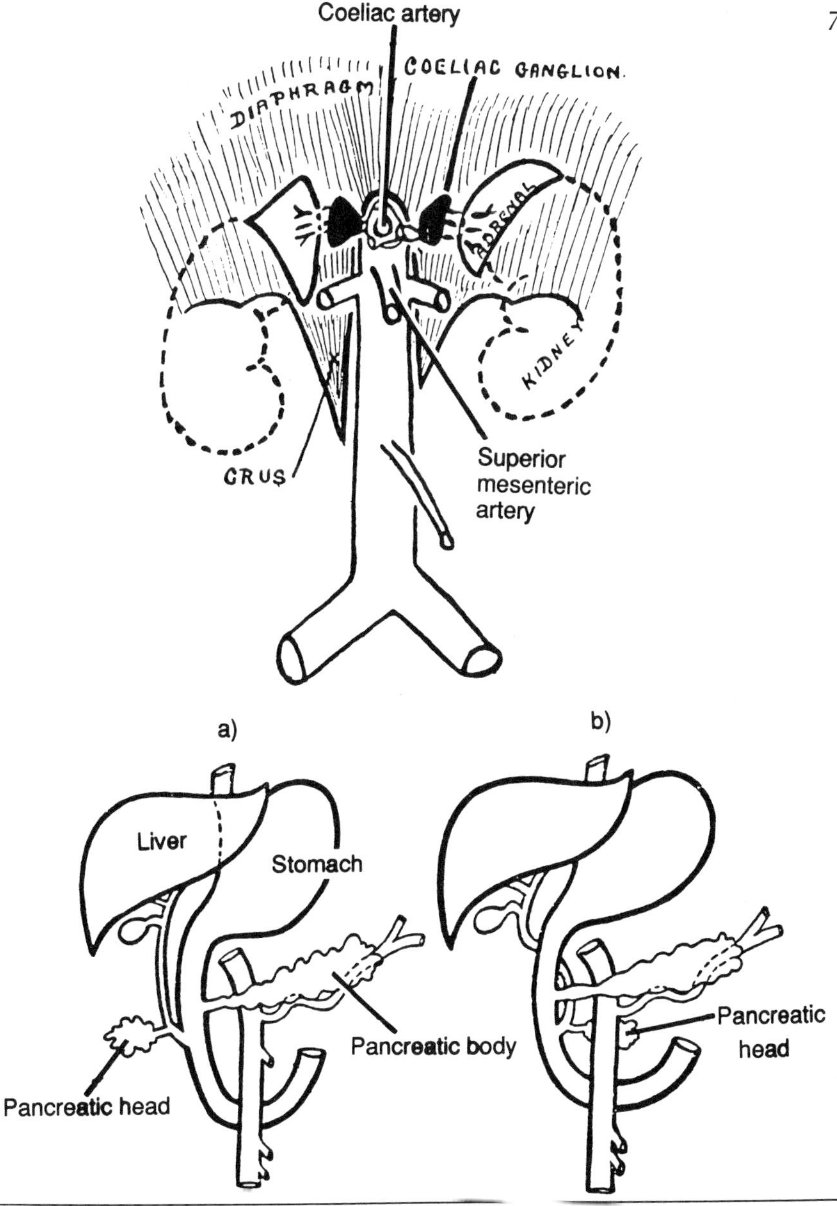

d: Showing the manner in which the coeliac artery, the blood pipe to the stomach, arrests the descent of the main part of the diaphragm, but not the crura.

e: The two buds of the pancreas (a) before and (b) after rotation.

The sketches were probably drawn by J.C.B. They are taken from Grant's article listed in Appendix 1, reference 3.

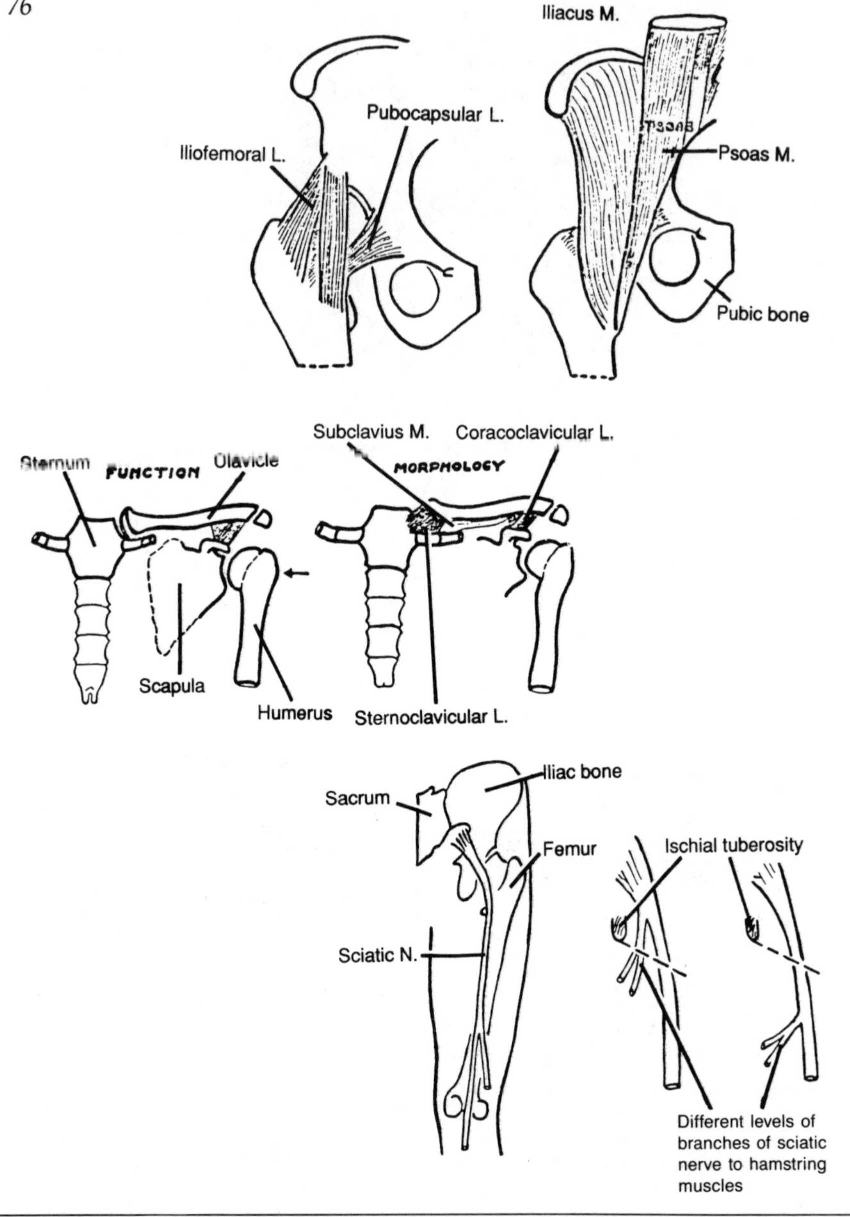

Anatomical relationships. University of Manitoba, 1927.

a: Ball-and-socket hip joint, showing supports of ligaments and two muscles.

b: Showing the arrangement from sternum to scapula, of structures to protect against stress: inter-articular disc, clavicle, coraco-clavicular ligament, subclavius muscle.

c: The sacrum, ilium and femur from behind. Muscles attached to the ischial tuberosity of the ilium are supplied by branches which leave the sciatic nerve on the same side, at variable levels.

at today's crowded meetings. However, the facts are precise, and Grant covers the subject with an air of confident authority reinforced by his innate modesty. "I am not," he disclaims, "one of those who believe they have a message which must at all costs be delivered to the world; neither am I one of those who are perpetually and profoundly dissatisfied with all present methods of teaching."

> As undergraduates we were taught the structure of the human body thoroughly and well. Like others I was, and am, influenced by the environment and by the traditions of the school which was my cradle, and I teach much after the fashion in which I was taught. I have, however, long felt that anatomy would have meant much more to me had I been led at an earlier stage of my career to appreciate more thoroughly a number of these general principles, which, as it is, have formulated themselves under the guidance of experience.
>
> It is by the application of principles (or generalizations) and by the correlation of facts that we try to guide and teach our students to think and to reason anatomically. I am not using the term "principles" in the platitudinous sense in which it is so often used. For example, I remember a certain teacher who in his lectures had a strong obsession for explaining at great length how certain conditions could be diagnosed from a careful study of the nature and distribution of referred pains; but, in his clinic this teacher never made mention of these pains. He struck me as being like one who is inconsistently a Christian on Sundays and a pagan on weekdays, for though he sang the praises of referred pains during lecture hours, he committed the sins of omission against them at all other times. As a teacher he was a failure.
>
> Not long ago a surgeon of some unmerited renown remarked to me that he saw no purpose in requiring students to commit to memory such useless details as the attachment of the adductor muscles of the thigh. I thoroughly agreed with him that the attachment of these muscles should not be committed to memory; I agreed that their attachments were, perhaps, of no great importance; but, at the same time I told him that we expected our students to know, not merely the attach-

ments, but also the nature of the attachments of muscles; whether they are fleshy or tendinous or aponeurotic. Our students appreciate such matters; they are, moreover, aware that if they could not answer such questions they would be liable to come to grief for displaying ignorance, not of origins and insertions, but of the first principles of anatomy.

Now this surgeon knew well that on the back of the femur there extends a rough line, the linea aspera; he knew that the rest of the shaft of the bone is smooth, but these points meant nothing to him. He was one of the many "Peter Bells" of whom Wordsworth said, "A primrose by a river's brim, a yellow primrose was to him, and it was nothing more." Of course, there are two possible causes for rough markings on a healthy bone. One is the site of an old epiphyseal line; the other, the attachment of fibrous tissue, be it tendon, ligament, fascia, dura mater, or the like. As the linea aspera is patently not an epiphyseal line, it must, by exclusion, be the site of attachment of fibrous tissue. And as the quadriceps femoris muscle monopolizes the smooth parts of the circumference of the shaft of the femur, the attachment of the adductors must, again by exclusion, be the linea aspera, and, therefore, must be aponeurotic. This has, at least, the following clinical significance: the femoral artery is separated from the profunda femoris artery by the adductor longus, and as these vessels lie close to the femur, it follows that it is the aponeurotic and not the fleshy portion of the adductor longus which divides these vessels from each other. Accordingly, the ragged end of a fractured femur, a gunshot wound, a stab, or a tumour involving one vessel is very liable to involve the other. Or, again, a surgeon performing an amputation through the thigh, having tied the femoral artery, will not require to grope about for the profunda femoris but will find it separated from the parent vessel only by the thickness of an aponeurosis.

The next part of the paper has several examples of the deductive method and some impressionable line drawings. The first shows the iliac bone, the head of the femur, and the ligaments of the joint in front, in one view, and in the next the psoas tendon in place, between the ligaments.

> Due to our erect posture, our line of gravity passes behind the hip joint, therefore the capsule of the hip joint is thickened in front, the thickening being known as the ilio-femoral ligament or the ligament of Bigelow. For the same reason, the excess of articular cartilage on the ball-like head of the femur is directed forwards. And while the lateral part of this exposed area is protected by the ilio-femoral ligament and the medial part by the pubo-capsular ligament, the intermediate part, which most requires support, which Nature did not ignore, has the tendon of the psoas muscle....

The whole femur, the iliac bone with a small part of the attached sacrum, and the "bare" sciatic nerve running from the sacro-iliac notch, to its division into the medial and lateral popliteal nerves illustrates an anatomical principle: branches of nerves to muscles leave the parent trunk from the side nearest to the muscle—in the case of the hamstrings, the medial side — but the level at which the branch leaves the parent nerve is variable.

Grant cites the case of a surgeon ("on another continent") who, while operating on the gluteal region, remarked as he worked that the sciatic nerve supplied no muscle in that region, whereupon he proceeded freely to expose the nerve on all sides. Had he reasoned that the lateral side of the sciatic nerve was the only safe side he would not have stripped the main trunk of the branches to the biceps and semitendinosus which, in this case, arose from the sciatic nerve much higher than usual. Elsewhere in the paper, exactly the same principle is demonstrated with the medial popliteal nerve and the median and radial nerves at the elbow.

He stresses that we do not try to memorize, but to understand. Another drawing illustrates how the morphology of the clavicle and its attachments protect the body after a fall on the shoulder.

He deals with the then young science of embryology as related to anatomy. He disagreed with the lavish amount of time allocated in some schools to embryology—"perhaps the youth and charm of this branch, rather than its utility, are responsible for the prolonged attentions devoted to it." He concentrated on those aspects of embryology having practical importance, especially the bile duct and pancreas. One diagram shows the developing pancreas as two buds, the head with a duct entering the common bile duct on the right of the duodenum, and tail with the accessory pancreatic duct on the left but in front of the portal vein. The next drawing shows the head of the pancreas after it has rotated through 180 degrees behind the duodenum to bring the portal vein to its permanent home, taking the common bile duct with it. "The two rudiments of the pancreas thus close upon the portal vein, much as one might close a book on a bookmark."

The final pictures in the embryology section are of the genito-urinary organs. One drawing shows the sex organ, testis or ovary, descending in front of the ureter while the kidney ascends, and the next the testis with the vas deferens and the ovary with "its duct", the Fallopian tube, in their final resting place, still in front of the ureter. He remarks that although the vas deferens develops from the Wolffian duct, and the uterine tube from the Mullerian duct, these are but names for two ducts which develop in the embryo, and which lie side by side throughout their course, until eventually one predominates in the male and the other in the female.

The final paragraphs in the paper reveal, in places almost poetically, Grant's burning desire to pass on the secrets of his teaching method so that his life's interest, human anatomy, will live.

> Briefly, then, these and such things run through and dominate our teaching of gross anatomy in the lecture theatre, in tutorial class and, as we pass daily from table to table, in the dissecting room. At times, we make an appeal to a principle or, it may be, to a consideration of function or, again, to some important clinical point. At another time an embryological or, it may be, a morphological explanation clears up an otherwise difficult point, and often our appeal is to the simple and obvious. Due regard is paid to the common and important variations in the human body, for each student is detailed to investigate all the cadavera in the rooms for some specified point, such as the number of notches in the spleen, the presence of accessory hepatic ducts, the variations in distribution of a certain nerve, vessel or tendon, and the like. In this way he becomes acquainted with the fact that no two

human beings are identical in construction. Each student, moreover, makes a careful dissection which, if of sufficient merit, is placed in our museum as a lasting record of his work. In the third and fourth year, a demonstration per week is devoted to the subject of applied anatomy, instruction in which subject is under the care of a practising surgeon who has special anatomical training.

In the teaching of anatomy there are four important elements—a student, a cadaver, a teacher and a sufficient amount of time. All else is subsidiary to these. In my experience, part-time assistants may be demonstrators, but for the most part, they are apt to be untrustworthy as teachers, and the function of imparting instruction we are not prepared to trust to their care.

Now, I am fully aware that the bare, the dry, the unadorned and unrelated facts evaporate from the memory as soon almost as the objects of study are withdrawn from the vision. It is my belief that one should not attempt the almost hopeless task of trying to commit to memory bald anatomical details, but the important relationships and facts should always be within certain and easy recall. I have tried to show how pictures of relationships may be summoned up so as again to become vivid and very real.

Grant returned to Winnipeg on 10 October 1958 for a special Convocation of the University of Manitoba in his honour. Dean Bell presented him to the Senate for the conferring of the degree of Doctor of Science, *honoris causa*.

The present Professor and head of anatomy at the University of Manitoba, Dr. T.V.N. Persaud points to the uniqueness and popularity of the textbook which sets it above all others.[7] He attributes this to Grant's reliance on logic, analysis and deduction as opposed to dry memory work. It is no wonder that, in a span of about fifty years, the book has been printed thirty times during its eight editions. The equally popular *Atlas*, first published in 1943, was also conceived in Manitoba, and many of the original specimens and drawings are still in the department. When Grant left Manitoba, his colleagues felt that they were "parting with a friend whose presence we would give much to retain."

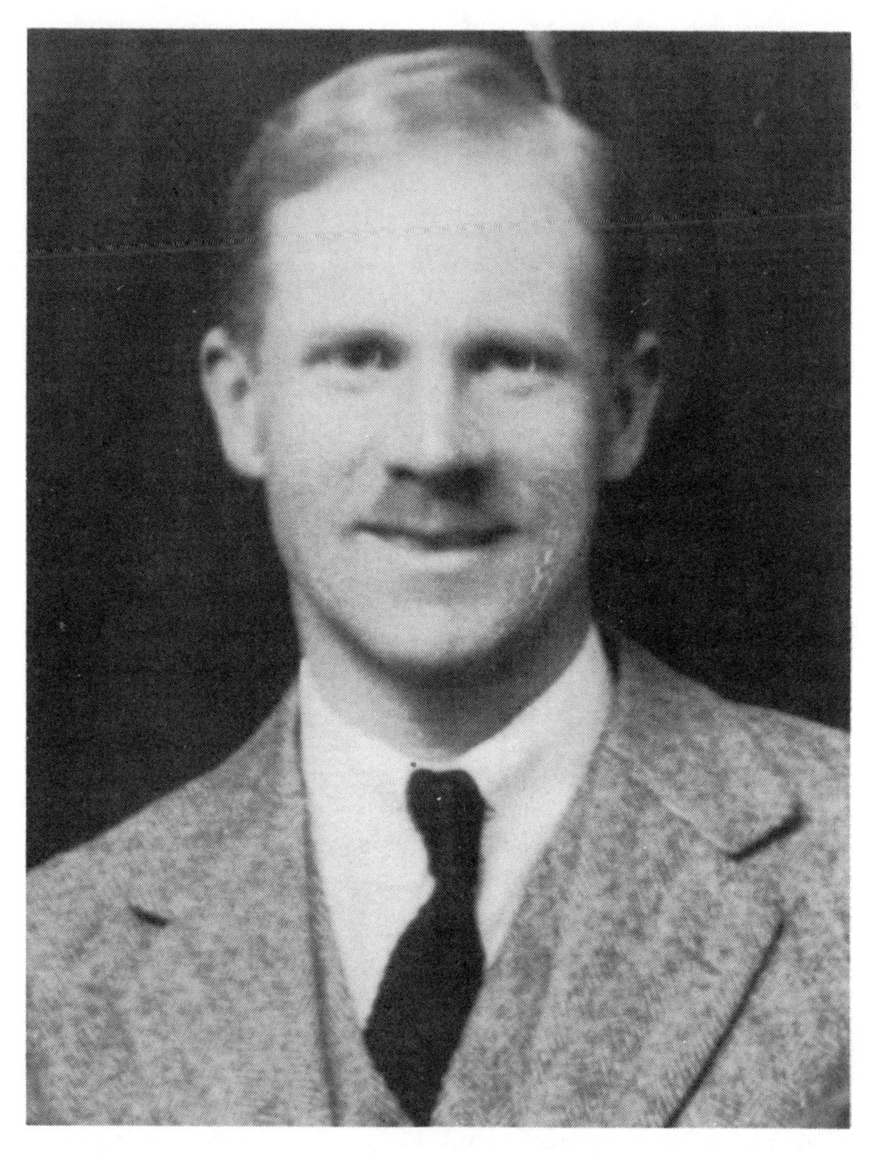

J.C.B. receiving degree of Doctor of Science, University of Manitoba.

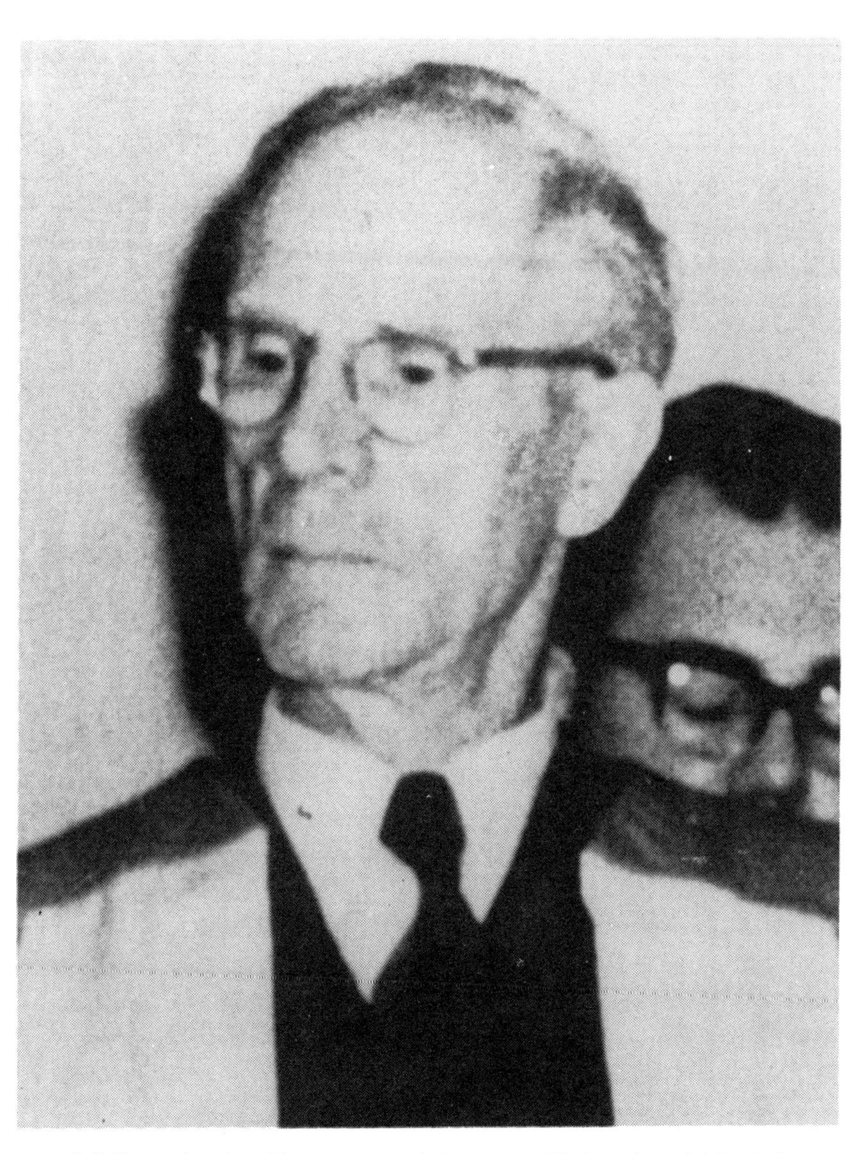

J.C.B. on leaving Department of Anatomy, University of Manitoba.

The teaching of normal histology was transferred from the department of pathology to the department of anatomy, a natural change which Grant and William Boyd, as Professor of Pathology, had no difficulty in effecting. Grant, courteous as always, acknowledged in his annual report the generous assistance he had received from Boyd when the move was made. Transfers of this sort between university departments are not always undertaken so amicably. No doubt the lasting camaraderie from student days of the principals and their marriages to sisters guaranteed a trouble-free reorganization.

The anatomy class consisted of about one hundred students and the course extended over two years. Because of a shortage of cadavers more than half the students had to dissect fetuses, neither "with zeal nor with relish". Each year students had to take three examinations, one written and two oral.

The size of the staff was small and consisted of the professor, one or two full-time appointments and a large number of honorary (unpaid) demonstrators. The department had two technicians who were responsible for the preparation of all teaching materials.

Grant's opinion of his students is as much a tribute to the respect and affection they held him in as to their innate good behaviour. Medical students do not as a rule suffer a poor teacher gladly. He wrote in one of his annual reports that he "would like to express the opinion that nowhere are there students who behave with more propriety or act with more consideration for their teachers than those working in this Department." Many senior students would return to the department at the end of the day to review their anatomy and to assist in the preparation of specimens for the museum.

Adam Little, a graduate of the class of 1942, later described Dr. Grant as a tall, sandy-haired Scotsman. "His manner is that of a modest, cultured and altogether successful man." To Little, Grant fitted Emerson's description of the type of man who is "relieved and gay when he has put his heart into his work and done his best." Grant was once asked what qualities he considered to be most valuable in a physician. Without hesitation he gave "sympathy and understanding for his patient, a high degree of moral integrity, and in case of difficulty or doubt, a readiness to consult a colleague".

When Grant left Winnipeg for Toronto a colleague mourned the departure not merely of the Professor of Anatomy, sad loss though it was, but also of a personality richly endowed with that elusive gift of charm, the humorous remark and the quizzical smile. It would not take Toronto long to discover how well it had done for itself.

Grant resigned his position in Manitoba at the end of July 1930. At the time, the British Medical Association was meeting in Winnipeg with the Canadian Medical Association. His departure was overshadowed by the activities of the moment. But after the convention the medical faculty in Winnipeg, in recognition of his teaching and of his interest in North American Indian anthropology, presented him with an oil painting by N. Grandmaison of See-Kee-Quatin, of Duck Lake, Sask., one of the braves who took part in the Riel Rebellion of 1885.

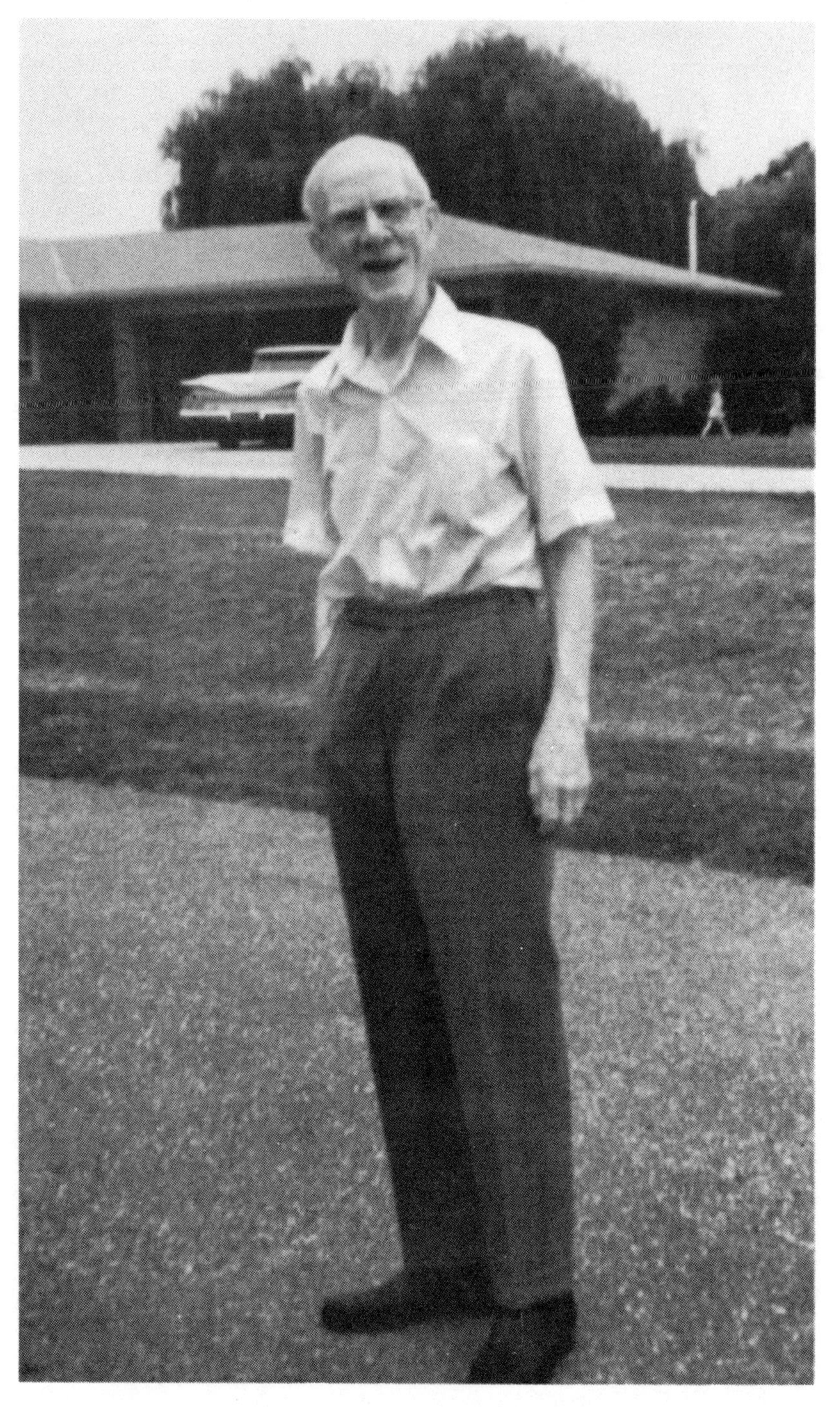

J.C.B. outside his house on Arjay Crescent, Toronto.

— Chapter 7 —

University of Toronto

GRANT succeeded J. Playfair McMurrich (1859—1939) as professor at Toronto. McMurrich, who had succeeded Alexander Primrose in 1907, was one of the most distinguished University of Toronto graduates the medical school had seen. His embryology text, *The Development of the Human Body,* was used in many parts of the world. Apart from his extensive anatomical writings, he was an accomplished biologist (PhD, Johns Hopkins University) and had been Professor of Biology at the Ontario Agricultural College at Guelph. He resigned from the Chair of the Department of Anatomy at the University of Michigan, which he had occupied after his appointment at Guelph, to return to Toronto. In 1930 he published *Leonardo Da Vinci, Anatomist,* at the request of the Carnegie Institute. The anatomy building into which Grant moved had been built in 1923 following the benefaction to the University of the Rockefeller Foundation. It was appropriately named the McMurrich Building.

As the Professor, Grant was strikingly different from McMurrich. McMurrich was the greater academician but Grant was the greater teacher. McMurrich allowed his students and staff to do their work in the manner of their own choosing. In consequence, some grasped the opportunity to do very little. Grant, on the other hand, kept close contact with his students, demonstrators, staff and artists, to ensure the work was thoroughly and accurately carried out. Some, particularly the demonstrators, rejoiced in the attention Grant gave to their studies. Others found the pressure not always conforming to their style of working.

Grant wrote: ''In 1930, I accepted an invitation to the Chair of Anatomy in the University of Toronto, and remained there until 1956. Thereupon, I was appointed Curator of the Anatomy Museum in the University.''

> In Toronto, my first objective was to create a museum, a teaching museum of anatomical material that would be used. It was so designed that the specimens were placed in four-sided jars, and set on revolving bases; hence, each specimen had four surfaces to present, each was specially illustrated and labelled. These the student, seated and with textbook or notes beside him, could study in comfort.

The late Ross G. MacKenzie was a member of the department for many years. His history draws a detailed picture of the department at that time.[1]

> The Grant days can only be described as exciting and stimulating. It was during this period that the department of anatomy was repeatedly voted by the graduating class as the best in the faculty for undergraduate teaching. Discipline was strict for both staff and students but there was never any indication that this engendered a feeling of resentment because the students were well aware that all activities in the department were directed in their interests.
>
> During the academic year three lectures were given each week by Professor Grant. These always dealt with the region under dissection in the laboratory. They were illustrated by sharp, accurate, line drawings that were never cluttered with minutiae but forcibly stressed the important features of the region under discussion.
>
> The students were required to spend approximately twelve hours each week dissecting in the gross anatomy laboratory where they were under the supervision of an adequate number of demonstrators. The laboratory was open from nine to five

every weekday throughout the session with the exception of Saturday when it closed at noon.

The embryology of individual organs was studied concurrently with their dissection. General embryology was taught by the department of zoology in the second premedical year.

Dr. Grant was responsible for the appointment of Arthur Ham as head of the section of histology. Just as Grant had brought an exciting approach to the teaching of gross anatomy, so Ham gave the teaching of histology a real ''lift'' as function and structure were inseparably linked. The course consisted of forty-seven lectures and lecture demonstrations and ninety-four hours of practical work.

During the McMurrich years, an excellent course was given in neuroanatomy by Eric Linell, brought into the department by McMurrich from the University of Manchester in England, until he transferred to the department of pathology as the first neuropathologist. It was continued by H.A. Cates in the early years of Grant's period. The course consisted of thirty-two lectures and thirty-two hours of laboratory work. During most of the Grant days the course was under the direction of Dr. Carlton Smith who brought it to a peak of perfection. He collected his lectures and demonstrations together in his *Basic Neuroanatomy*, first published in 1961 with several reprints and finally a second edition in 1971.[2]

The anatomical museum which was incomplete and which had received very few new additions over the years was, under Dr. Grant's direction, rapidly expanded in quantity and quality. It was redesigned to aid the students in their studies. Thus great attention was given to the mounting and presentation of the specimens in order to obtain a maximum degree of clarity for the viewer. The specimens were prepared by the staff under the careful scrutiny of Dr. Grant, and dissections of merit by the students were frequently added to the permanent display. Grant, knowing that any success the *Atlas* might achieve depended on the illustrations, enlisted talented artists. Dorothy Chubb and Nancy Joy executed most of the illustrations. Eila Hopper, already committed as second-in-command to Maria Wishart, the department head, was able to set aside time for only one illustration, the pelvis, which because of its artistry and

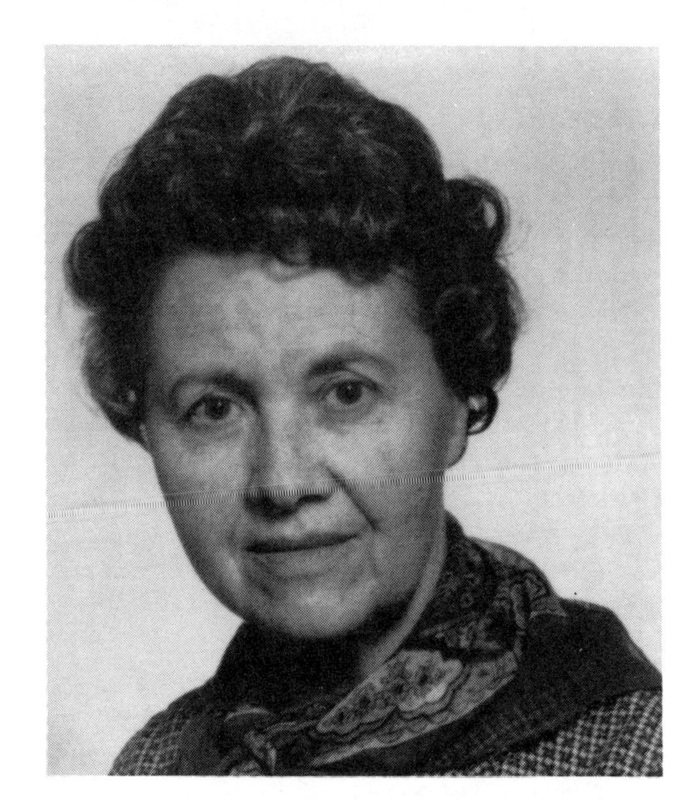

Dorothy Chubb

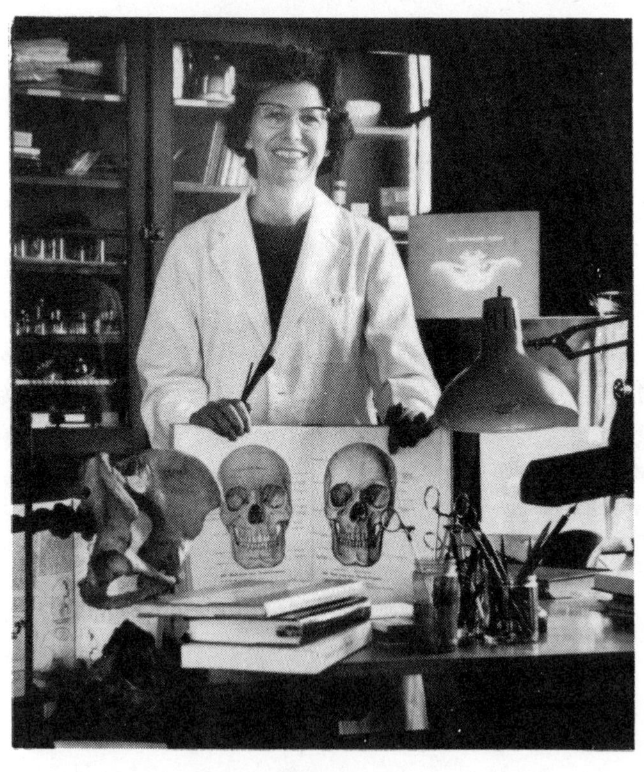

Nancy Joy

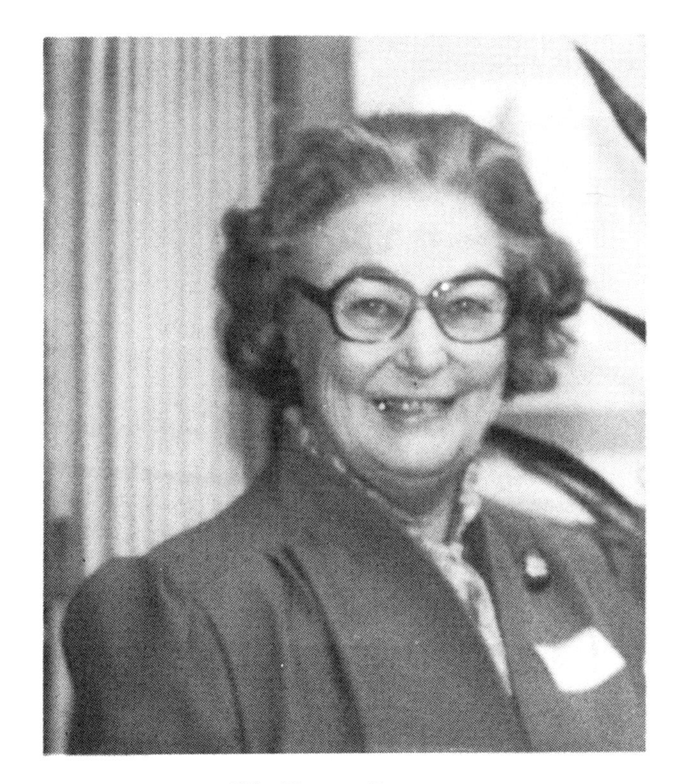

Eila Hopper Ross

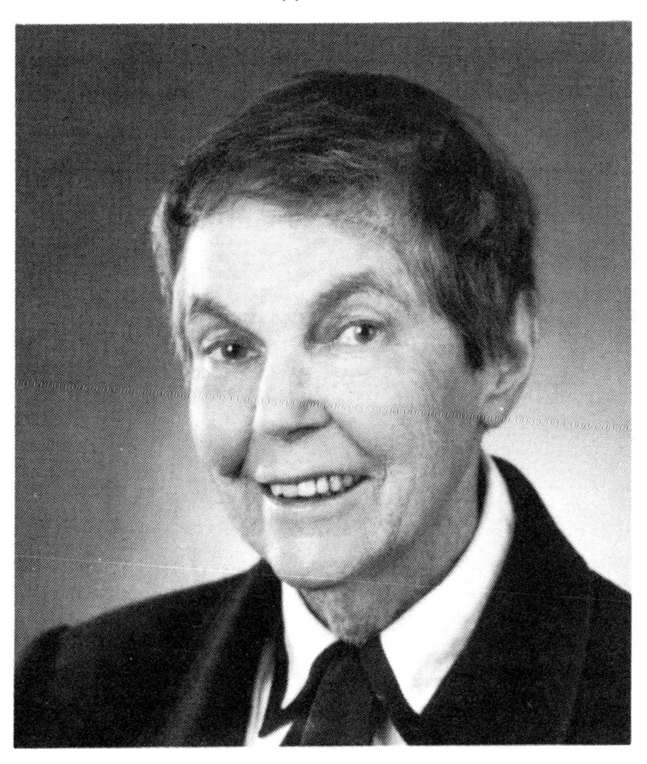

Elizabeth Blackstock

sense of depth was one of Grant's favourites. Elizabeth Blackstock drew a number of cross-sectional views of the limbs and Marguerite Drummond some pen-and-ink drawings of the anatomy of certain blood vessels. Grant's insistence on accuracy in every tiny detail during all stages of development of a picture made severe demands on the patience of the artists. The museum, now appropriately known as the Grant Museum, contains many of the specimens which are to be found illustrated in Grant's *Atlas of Anatomy*.

Mrs. Dorothy Chubb worked with Dr. Grant on the *Atlas* from 1940 to 1972. The last years were spent on the sixth edition, published in 1972. Mrs. Chubb had been married for two years when Grant first asked her to work for him. She recalls her first contact with Dr. Grant:

To David Christie

My old friend - pupil - and the brother of my Catriona.

15th May 1973. J C Boileau Grant

Inscription in a copy of the 6th edition of the Atlas of Anatomy, *2nd Asian edition, a few months before J.C.B. died.*

> I had heard that when Dr. Grant succeeded the gentle Dr. McMurrich as Professor of Anatomy he was a hard taskmaster with boundless nervous energy, whipping his staff into shape out of their previous easy-going ways and with a quick temper directed at erring students in the dissecting room. Reluctant, but thinking that perhaps I could manage a few drawings, I went to see him. He divulged his plan for producing an anatomy atlas; when I asked timidly how many illustrations there would be he replied, ''About five hundred.''
>
> I played for time and in February 1941 began working for him on the first edition of the *Atlas*, stating that I would do my best but could not be pressured. This rule he assiduously followed.

In the secluded atmosphere of the anatomy building Dorothy was installed in a room overlooking Queen's Park, sedulously guarded from interruptions. She was paid monthly on an hourly basis by the Williams and Wilkins Company, the future publishers of the *Atlas*. One of her staunch friends was Charlie Storton, who with Dr. Grant carefully prepared the specimens from which she worked. The process they developed is described in the Preface to the *Atlas of Anatomy*.

Charles Storton — Charlie — was engaged by Grant when he came to Toronto. Charlie was a lad of seventeen interested in developing a career in an unusual field in which he could make his mark. He knew nothing of work in a department of human anatomy when he arrived, and he had never encountered a man quite like Grant. He came near to giving it all up because of Grant's compulsive fussiness, but as his knowledge increased Grant gave him more responsibility until he had complete technical and administrative charge of the dissecting room and became indispensable to his Chief. Perhaps his most demanding and important job was the mounting of the specimens for the Museum in glass jars and sealing the lids. Grant's habit of removing the specimens from the jars to teach a class exasperated Charlie. The specimens dried out, became discoloured and misshapen, and Charlie saw his labours being squandered. His remedy was to seal the lids with a cement so tough that not even the professor could remove them. Charlie Storton worked with Grant for forty-nine years. Late in his career he took holy orders. Rev. Charles Storton is kept busy in his congregation in suburban Toronto

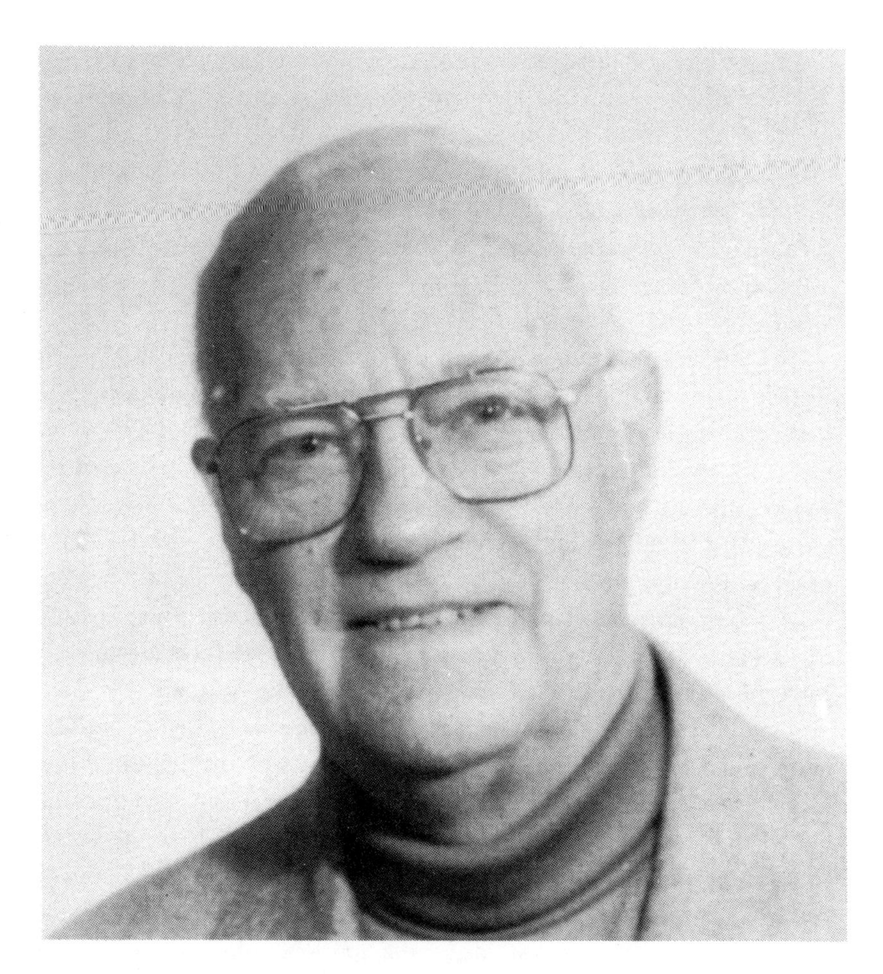

Rev. Charles Storton

but remains Charlie to those who know him.

In 1943 it was arranged for Dorothy to visit the publishers in Baltimore to learn if or how the reproduction of her drawings could be improved. Later, early in 1945, as Dr. Grant was unfolding his future plans for the *Atlas*, she had to tell him that she was expecting a baby in June and would be leaving. He received this startling blow gallantly, and after a pause quietly said, "I am glad you are going to have a family." So Dorothy became a homebody bringing up two little girls in whom John and Catriona took a lasting, affectionate interest. Later on the Grants were guests at Patricia Chubb's wedding. Throughout those years Dorothy did some illustrating for John at home.

In September 1969 she felt free to return to the old stomping ground, as John had patiently wanted her to do for many years. She was duly ensconced in the new Medical Sciences Building. After the 6th edition of the *Atlas* was published in 1972 she kept in touch with visits to the Grants at their home. When John was undergoing treatment for his cancer at the Princess Margaret Hospital she visited him there with Catriona.

"The years I spent working on the *Atlas of Anatomy* with Dr. John Grant," she said, "were filled with respect and growing affection for this remarkably dedicated and exacting master of human anatomy. His patience in clarifying a structure I was endeavouring to portray, his insistence on anatomical accuracy, my inherent perfectionism (the bane of my life at times) and our respect for each other's territory, made for a harmonious collaboration to achieve results satisfactory to both of us.

"As I knew him he was always a kind and courteous gentleman, most generous to me, a champion of my work and considerate of my home obligations—a friend of my family."

Nancy Joy's career as a medical artist began as a student in the four-year fine art programme at the Ontario College of Art, graduating in 1942. But her desire was to become a medical artist. So she attended courses with the Toronto medical students on anatomy, histology, neuroanatomy, embryology and pathology. She received no degree or credit because there was none to receive. But that was no obstacle to her almost thirty-year association as artist-illustrator to Grant.

Nancy recalls that, although there were eight female medical students in a class of 100 when she began her anatomy studies, Grant always addressed the assembled group with a cheery, "Good morning, gentlemen!"

After a few years at Toronto, Nancy went to the University of Illinois, Chicago, to continue her studies. She returned to Toronto to work with Dr. Grant but in 1956 she took a position as medical illustrator at the University of Manitoba where she was promoted to Assistant Professor of Medical Illustration in the Faculty of Medicine. In 1962 she returned to Toronto for the second time to be Professor and Chairman of the Department of Art as Applied to Medicine at the university. Through Nancy Joy's efforts a degree-granting programme was approved, leading to a Bachelor of Science in Art as Applied to Medicine (BSc.AAM).

For the first two years of the three year programme the AAM students study side by side with the medical students and write the same exams. Because of their depth of training, some graduates of the programme have filled positions in teaching hospitals, while others have served the needs of publishers, pharmaceutical companies, authors and individual medical specialists.

Such were Dorothy Chubb and Nancy Joy, the two pillars upon which Grant built the *Atlas*.

Through his textbooks Grant made an indelible impression on the teaching of anatomy throughout the world. The testimonials he received from the Canadian and American associations of anatomy point to the high esteem in which he was held by anatomists everywhere and by his former colleagues and students in those universities which were fortunate enough to have secured his appointment: Manitoba, Toronto and California at Los Angeles.

Grant was highly regarded by European anatomists. In the William Boyd Library of the Academy of Medicine in Toronto there is a framed engraving of a Wirsung dissection of 1642 showing for the first time the anatomy of the pancreatic ducts. On the back Grant has written over his signature, "One of the last reproductions it will be possible to obtain from the now worn-out plate of the discovery of the pancreatic ducts. A gift from Tullio Terni, successor of Vesalius of Padua, when we entertained him in Toronto."

When he considered leaving active teaching in Toronto, Grant said, "The time comes, you know," his eyes twinkling, "for the old horses to be put out to grass. The new head of the department, Dr. Duckworth, has very kindly not only given me free rein in the grass but a stable as well"—as Curator of the anatomy museum.

Between the walls of his basement stall in the anatomy building,

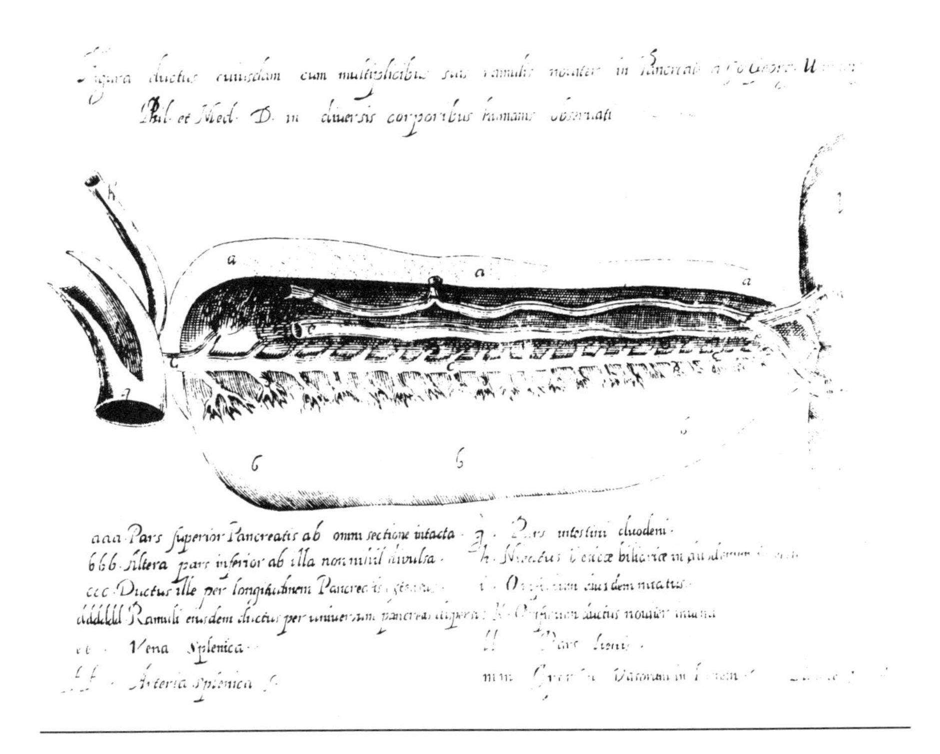

"One of the last reproductions it will be possible to obtain from the worn-out plate of the discovery of the pancreatic ducts. A gift from Tullio Terni, successor of Vesalius of Padua when we entertained him in Toronto." This is the inscription by Grant on the back of the picture mount. The discoverer was Johann Georg Wirsung (1600-1643) when he was prosector to Johann Vesling (1598-1649), professor of anatomy and botany at Padua. "Wirsung's discovery ... is recorded only on a single anatomical sheet of 1642, now very rare." (Singer, C. and Underwood, E.A.. A Short History of Medicine. *Oxford. Clarendon Press. 2nd. ed., 1962, p.516.) The engraving given to Grant, of which this illustration is a photograph, is, presumably, from the original plate.*

Grant was as busy as ever after his retirement. He revised the textbooks he had written over the course of his teaching years. ''Books are like people,'' he said. ''You have to feed plants and people—and books are the same. They have to be kept up to date.''

Asked about the highlights of his teaching years, he said, ''Well, everything is highlight. Summers and winters — why, there are highlights all the time!'' A good description of the lively life that began in Edinburgh some seventy years before. ''I thought anatomy was an essential step to surgery,'' he said about his early postgraduate training, ''but I kept on with it for four years. The World War came and after that I got the chair in anatomy in Winnipeg — so I stayed.''

Grant was not above learning from his surgical colleagues. Gordon Fahrni (now aged one-hundred-and-six) was established in surgical practice in Winnipeg when Grant arrived. Shortly afterwards Fahrni asked ''Grantie'', as he called him, to attend in the operating room during the removal of a thyroid gland. Fahrni believed there was very little anastomosis between the superior and inferior thyroid arteries. He had discussed the question with Grant over a cadaver in the anatomy department and was anxious to pursue the matter *in vivo* with him. Grant may have felt obliged to answer the summons to the operating room by a more senior colleague, but his willingness to do so was in keeping with his conviction that the role of an anatomist was in the assisting of clinicians.

While he was in Winnipeg, Grant became engrossed with the anthropology of the North American Indian although ''it was only a hobby.'' He explained that ''nothing was being done in Canada about the measurements and blood groupings of the Indians. I suggested the idea in Ottawa, and so, I was sent out.'' Without a doubt the work was difficult and physically arduous.

''You've got to learn the technique,'' he went on. ''You've got to have interpreters and much more. And you can't just walk in, then measure them, of course.'' One tribe in 1922 somehow got the impression that he was there to measure them *and* to take a census for the next war. ''They just disappeared into the woods!'' he recalled with a chuckle.

In 1934, flying from Waterways at the end of steel to Fort Resolution on Great Slave Lake, Grant spent the summer in the Mackenzie River basin to obtain further anthropological data on the Athabascan stock of Indians. It was in the middle of one of these expeditions to the Northwest Territories that Grant was notified that he had been offered the chair of anatomy at Toronto. "I still don't know how they found me," he confessed. "I was somewhere out in the woods, going up to visit some Indians on horseback when I got the telegram. I had a choice of giving it up, hurrying back and spoiling the summer — or taking my chances. Well, I decided to go on. And when the time came, I managed to find a plane somewhere, and fly out to Edmonton and take a train to Toronto."

This was in 1930. "Toronto is a pretty city," he reflected not long after his arrival, "if they don't fill up all the ravines. It has a lot of natural beauty. And one likes the people." It wasn't long before the Grants acquired a cottage on the north shore of Lake Ontario where Grant tried to keep the lake from swallowing the property. "The water is a very intelligent thing, you know," he warned. "Each summer I find another way of getting around it — and the water wins every year." In the winter Catriona was fond of skating and Grant was enchanted watching her as she cut her figures on the ice.

Among his trophies were a self-winding watch, a summer "sun couch", a pair of rugged buffalo book-ends and a handsome letter opener that roughly resembles a scalpel. These had been given him "with affection and gratitude from students past and present". They were the tangible expressions of the legend of the teacher during his quarter-century at Toronto.

On his retirement a varsity journal revealed "his little-known talents for mouth-organs and monkeyshines, which have enlivened the charmed circle of his friends."

Students are not known for handing out undeserved compliments about their teachers, most of whom are soon forgotten when their time is up. But a few, like Grant, are fiercely championed by those who were so fortunate as to sit at their feet.

"I have never been so impressed by the integrity of a professor," one student said of Grant. "I have never had more respect for a teacher. But why? I don't know why!" Perhaps it was because he was the only senior professor who never missed a class party. Perhaps because he locked himself in his office for fifteen minutes before each lecture to review once more a topic he had already delivered many times. It may have been because, when a student came to ask him for a recommendation for a scholarship, he set aside an hour to become acquainted with him.

"A fantastic character" was the opinion of another student. "His actions, his voice, his phenomenal patience, his dry wit, his surprising and pleasing little idiosyncrasies added up to a lecturer that we will never see replaced."

"He tried to make us reason by basic principles," another recalled. "When he came to the lab, you never forgot anything he said."

Lectures and labs were not the only focus of his students' admiration. They were equally awed by his "tremendous knowledge" of anything to do with anatomy, and his work in criminology involving the identification of human bones added piquancy to the legend; they heard he had refused to sit for an official portrait and were pleased by his disdain to conform; they struggled to keep up with him as he took the stairs three at a time; they sat through at least three lectures before they knew what he was driving at, then patience brought its own reward. Respect, tinged with a little fear, greeted him as he swept into the classroom. "The last of the gentlemen," they said. "Above all an imperialist, a Scotsman, and an Edinburgh man who never forgot it."

To his staff he was "The Chief" and "the greatest living practical anatomist." But for successions of Medsmen who cut up their cadavers under J.C. Boileau Grant's instruction, he was, quite simply, what he most wanted to be — an anatomy teacher.

W.D. Stevenson, who became head of neurosurgery at Dalhousie University, recalls:

> I was a student of Grant from 1932 to 1934 at Toronto, which was soon after his arrival from Manitoba. My demonstrator in anatomy was Harry Botterell (a 1930 graduate of University of Manitoba). He was beginning his postgraduate work in surgery with a period of study in anatomy, a common prerequisite at that time. This was mainly due to the importance of anatomy as a subject in the Canadian fellowship primary examinations. Dr. Botterell invited me to study anatomy with him in his garret room in Hart House in the evenings. We were both privileged to sit in special classes which Dr. Grant gave at regular intervals for the demonstrators and a few lucky students. And what a teacher Dr. Grant was! The anatomical drawings which he could build up on the blackboard, layer upon layer of coloured chalk, were almost unforgettable (except at examination time), and he always seemed to be able to tell a story or make some comment which would engrave the subject on your memory.

> For example, in this way he used the tiny auricular branch of the vagus nerve (also called Arnold's nerve) which supplies part of the external ear canal. Dr. Grant ensured our recollection of it by calling it the alderman's nerve, after aldermen in the old town councils in England who, to deflect the opposition in debate, would sometimes scratch inside the ear canal with the little finger to induce vomiting!
>
> Dr. Grant's high-pitched, squeaky voice made him a common target for students' take-off at the annual Daffydil Night — the Christmas concert — in Hart House theatre. There was many a spoof of his characteristic teaching ways, but I cannot recall one which was anything but kindly towards him, as he was almost universally liked by his pupils. I will always remember him as a true inspiration. He was a gentleman, kindly, and in his dedication always in pursuit of excellence.

In the very first lecture in anatomy, Grant admonished his students to view the dead in the dissecting room with propriety and decorum. He next exhorted them to keep their knives sharp for dissection. If he discovered a blunt knife among a student's instruments he was liable to throw it on the floor. He devoted several pages in the *Method* to the importance of a sharp knife and the correct technique for sharpening it. Another tip to make the dissection a work of art was to discard veins, leaving the arteries uncluttered and easy to see. "Where there is an artery there is always a vein," he would say.

A graduate of 1959 has recorded fond memories from his student days in the 1950s when he was in one of the last classes taught by Grant.

> At that time Professor Grant was already a legend; by the time of the first lecture, I was already duly impressed that I was privileged to be in the presence of such a famous person. Interesting to say, he was not the Great Communicator in the present-day understanding of that word. That is, I never did manage to understand more than half the words he spoke! Fortunately, his textbook and atlas followed closely his annual course of lectures.
>
> His whole bearing as a professor revealed his sense of duty and devotion to his teaching, furtherance of his profession and

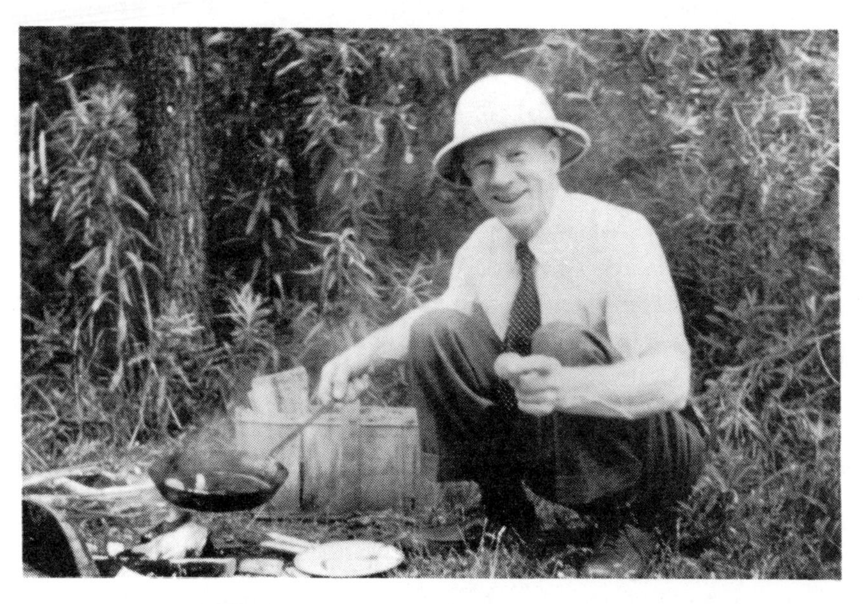

J.C.B. at his Pickering property (site of present nuclear power station), circa 1960.

> pursuit of excellence. He conveyed a sense of the theatrical. At ten past nine the amanuensis opens the lecture room door and J.C.B. Grant enters in professorial gown, the red hair a little askew and, to the accompaniment of a somewhat mumbled lecture, he proceeds to fill the blackboard with his famous sketches.
>
> To make sure we did our work he conducted seminars at the end of each week to expose our weaknesses. He also made a point of paying random visits to the anatomy lab.
>
> So it was when one day we were gathered around the demonstrator at a table in the lab. Being short of stature, I was in the back of the circle and could not see the subject well. Suddenly, I was physically lifted up and pushed forward toward the table. Somewhat annoyed, I turned around and looked the Professor smack in the face! "Don't be shy, get a good look," or words to that effect came from the Professor. He was an exemplary man.[3]

Grant had the knack of reducing anatomical jargon to plain English the beginner could understand. The spatial relationships of one structure to another are described by the anatomist in terms such as medial, lateral, superior, inferior, posterior and anterior, concepts some students at first find difficult. On one occasion the course of the radial nerve above and below the elbow was under discussion. Dr. Grant asked the student how he would describe the direction of the nerve. After much humming and hawing on the part of the student, Dr. Grant said, "Come, come, come, Mr. Bell-Irving, does it go round and round and round, or does it go straight down, or does it go around and then straight down?"[4]

Dr. Grant left an unforgettable impression on W. Robert Harris.[5]

> I was fortunate in that I had demonstrated anatomy and histology for a year which, of course, increased my respect and affection for this remarkable man. While his demeanour seemed at first somewhat stern and forbidding, we soon discovered he was a warm-hearted person who would go to any length to help us. I particularly recall asking him to review the first scientific paper I wrote. In one hour he taught me more about the proper use of English and the origin of many words commonly used in medicine than I could have learned in a year by myself.

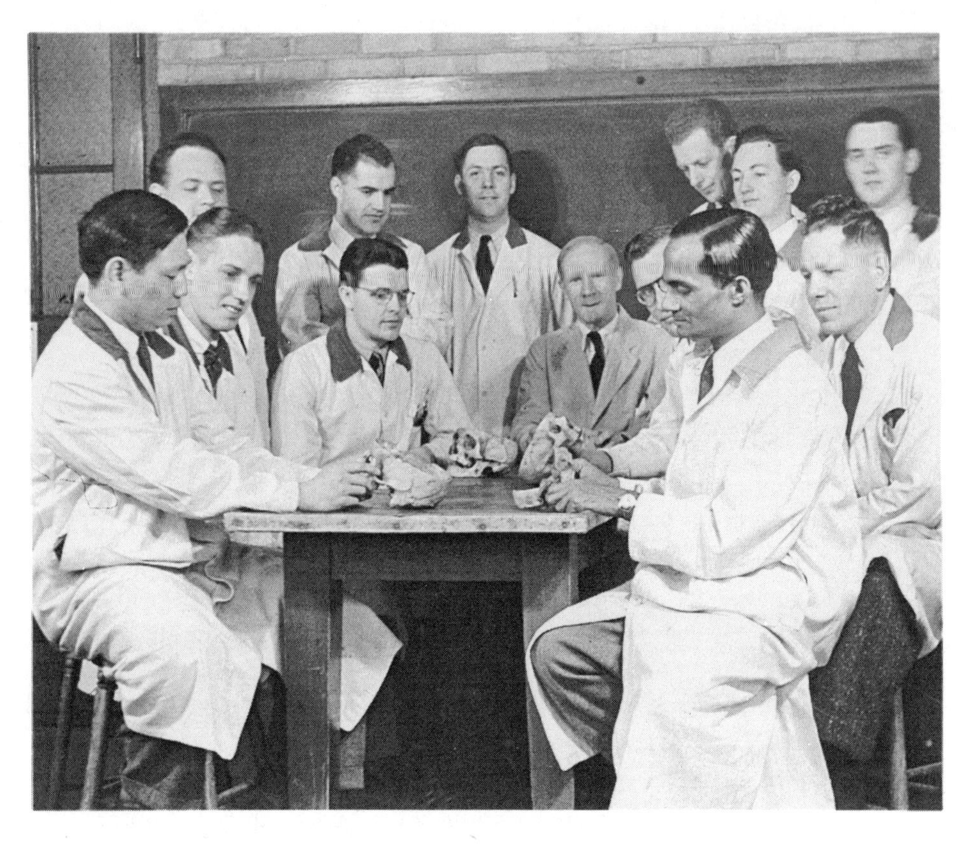

J.C.B. with anatomy demonstrators, Toronto, 1947-1948. Standing, left to right: John Hay, Bruce Wells, Keith Nancekivell, Harold Tovell, Unknown, John Callaghan. Sitting, left to right: Unknown, Jack McLister, Gordon Beattie, J.C.B., Hertz Rotenberg (partly concealed), Unknown (foreground), John Posnakoff. Subsequent careers of some of the demonstrators shown: Gordon Beattie (d.1986), head of general surgery, Ottawa Civic Hospital; Bruce Wells FRCSC, surgical staff, Oakville-Trafalgar Hospital, Ontario; Harold Tovell, obstetrics and gynaecology, New York City; Hertz Rotenberg, senior Ear, Nose and Throat specialist, USAAF; John Callaghan, cardiothoracic surgeon, Edmonton, Alberta; Keith Nancekivell, general surgeon, Thunder Bay, Ontario.

There can hardly be a doctor who, on looking back, fails to be thankful for the time Grant spent with his students. Surgeons, to whom human anatomy is fundamental to their practice, are perhaps more vocal than their non-surgical colleagues in their admiration of Grant.

Dr. James W. McGillivray, now in surgical practice in Collingwood, Ontario, was a first-year student in anatomy in 1949.

> I had never seen anyone draw with both hands before, and never could I have imagined that anyone could reproduce those anatomical pictures so accurately and with such great regularity. I found him very frightening in a strange way although it may have been the fact that I was a nervous youth and he was a great professor.
>
> He was a great stickler for correct pronunciation and, as would be natural for an anatomist, he had a special interest in the word "dissect". He pointed out to us early on that it was not pronounced "dye-sect", for that would be from the Greek and would mean cut in two; but rather it was from the Latin "dis" with the same pronunciation as disseminate, dissociate, and disintegrate, and that it meant spreading....
>
> As everyone knows, the "King's English" is the best spoken English. At that time (1949) one would have taken for granted that the prime model was King George VI himself. In his Christmas Day message to the Empire, His Majesty used the word dissect and used it, naturally, in the proper way, as Professor Grant had instructed us. Grant could scarcely wait until the lecture began to point this out to us. I have never forgotten this even though I have forgotten some of the other things that he taught us.
>
> The other most unforgettable lecture was on the perineum. He described Colles' fascia and how it contained "things" within this particular pouch or envelope. He gave the example of a boy who was walking on top of a fence when he lost his balance and fell astride the fence. Dr. Grant, with beautiful timing, brought his outstretched index and middle fingers down astride his pointer as if it were the boy falling with his legs akimbo. The gasp in the lecture theatre was more than merely audible; the sickening feeling was shared by all who had ever imagined or experienced a similar injury.

Professor Grant was always very strict about proper dignity and decorum; he mentioned what a privilege it was to learn our anatomy by dissecting the dead. He was in a great fury one day when he caught one of my classmates skipping with a length of some poor fellow's small intestine.

He had a gentle side too. I felt that at the bell-ringer examinations he was quite a reasonable questioner, although it was with trepidation that I approached his station.

The demonstrators — ten or twelve at a time — were young graduated physicians who were taken on, without salary, to help undergraduate students with their dissections; the position was unpaid except for veterans who received a nominal sum through the federal Department of Veterans' Affairs. A demonstrator, however, applied for the position knowing there was no better way to prepare for the inevitable anatomy questions in the later specialty examinations for surgery; few intended to follow careers in anatomical research or teaching. Demonstrators struggled to keep a few pages ahead of their students while Grant gave them regular tutorials which took the form, in fact, of oral examinations. He was not pleased if a demonstrator was slow in answering his questions, but the demonstrators realized Grant was doing it for his own good as well as for the students.

At that time, Eaton's Santa Claus parade led by trumpeters was held on a Saturday morning about a week before Christmas. The fanfare could be heard a long time before the parade arrived. The procession started a little before ten o'clock in the morning on College Street, not far from the university buildings. The last lecture of the week was given on Saturday at nine o'clock. Grant opened his lecture by saying that "at the first sound of the trumpets the class will be dismissed." True to his word, at a quarter to ten the members of the class fled to the parade to relive their childhood fantasies.

A demonstrator once asked Grant at a certain pause in a tutorial if he had ever smoked. Dr. Grant replied in his puckish way, "Oh, yes, lots of things; pine needles, tea leaves and so on." He did not enlarge on the theme, but the enquirer was left with a vision of the cold and wet soldier in the trenches seeking a little warmth and comfort, or the anthropologist in the Canadian north desperately trying to keep black flies and mosquitos at bay. In fact, he did smoke cigarettes at some time in his life, as a family photograph of the 1930s reveals. The picture was taken before the connection between smoking and lung cancer had been statistically established by Doll and Bradford Hill.[6] Grant would have been aware of Doll's work when, perhaps out of a sense of guilt, he finessed his student's question. The cancer that ended his life arose, paradoxically, in the trachea, a site not generally believed to be vulnerable to cancer in smokers, unlike lung and larynx.

When, in 1947, I went to London to take the primary examination for the fellowship of the Royal College of Surgeons of England, Professor Harris confronted me in the anatomy oral. He questioned me on a number of preserved anatomical specimens which gave me no trouble. In answer to his inquiry I told him that I had studied anatomy in Toronto. "Ah, yes," he murmured appreciatively, "Grant. No wonder you know it." When I recounted this story to Grant a shadow of a smile passed fleetingly across his face to acknowledge his pleasure, although by that time he must have known that his fame had spread across the continents.

Grant's style in the lecture theatre was formal even by the standards of the 1930s. "I was a student of Dr. Grant's in his anatomy classes at the University of Toronto in 1932 and 1933. His lectures were superb and very formal. He always wore an academic gown in his classes and always said 'good morning' to the class when he came in. I do not think we had another teacher in the Faculty of Medicine who ever wore an academic gown when giving his lectures. I did like this custom as it reflected the British tradition. We seem to have had relatively few such magnificent teachers in more recent years."[7]

It was the *Winnipeg Tribune* which, on 27 August 1936, six years after Grant had left Winnipeg for Toronto, reported:

> "M.O. AIDED WOUNDED CAPTAIN, GREETS HIM AS LORD STANLEY."
>
> Twenty-two years ago the Germans shelled the blue-blooded Grenadier Guards at Railway Wood and blasted the First Battalion of that proud regiment with high explosives and a land mine. A medical officer of the First Battalion staff found the captain badly wounded and carried him back to a dressing station on the Menin Road.

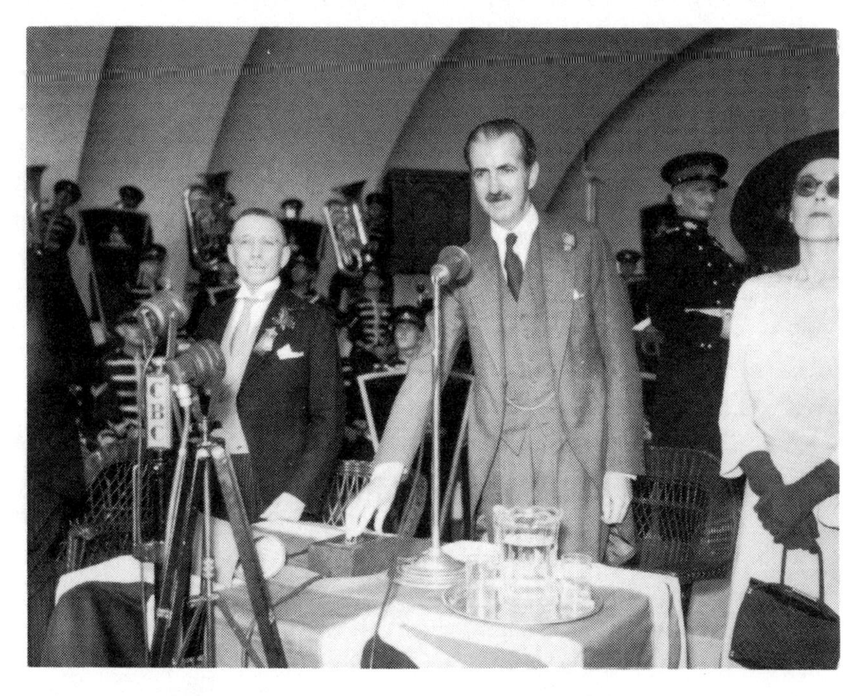

Lord Stanley opening the Canadian National Exhibition in Toronto in 1936 (Courtesy Canadian National Exhibition Archives, Toronto).

> For the first time in twenty years the captain and the doctor met again. To-day at the Royal York, the Captain, E.M.C. Stanley, and Dr. J.C.B. Grant talked over again the tragedy of Railway Wood and the years before, when they had known each other in the company mess.
>
> Added importance to their meeting is due to the fact that Capt. Stanley is Lord Stanley, who opened the CNE. And Dr. Grant is Prof. J.C.B. Grant, head of the Department of Anatomy, at the University of Toronto.[8]

The impression left with one student of the early 1960s of Grant in his declining years is of a black-coated, stooped figure arriving a little forlornly at his museum — a picture hard for any earlier student to imagine who knew him in his navy blue overcoat, ram-rod erect as befitted a Guard's officer.

Chapter 8

UCLA

"IN 1961-1962, I was invited to be Visiting Professor of Anatomy in the University of California, at Los Angeles (UCLA). This I accepted. This invitation has been extended annually and accepted for the last nine years. In my second year there the students were so generous as to dedicate to me their annual yearbook, *Meducla*."

C.H.Sawyer, now Emeritus Professor, was the chairman of the anatomy department when Grant started teaching at UCLA.

> Grant was with us (he writes) for eight years in the 1960s and a year in 1970. As always, he was revered by students and staff alike. The *Meducla* number dedicated to Dr. Grant was the 1965 issue; I am enclosing a xerox copy of the students' statement of dedication and the accompanying portrait of Dr. Grant.
>
> Another book with a special tribute to Dr. Grant was by the medical artist, May Lesser, entitled *The Art of Learning Medicine*.[1] Mrs. Lesser accompanied a class of medical students through their four years of medical school and described the experience in a book of her etchings....
>
> In our corridor of exhibits we have a skeleton of a young infant mounted in the upright position. Two ladies were

> looking at this show case as Dr. Grant and a student walked down the hall. When he came opposite them he asked the student in a voice loud enough for the ladies to hear, ''Did you know that that is the skeleton of George Washington as a baby?'' The ladies looked at the skeleton and at each other and one of them was heard to exclaim, ''I wonder why it is not in the Smithsonian.''

At the ceremony of dedication of *Meducla* a medical student paid this tribute:

> It is a difficult task to write a one-page tribute to seventy-nine years of a man's life. The gentleman's picture on the opposite page is J.C. Boileau Grant, author, professor, researcher, anatomist and physician. He came to UCLA four years ago as Professor Emeritus from the University of Toronto. All the students currently enrolled in the medical school have learned anatomy under his tutelage. Dr. Grant is a teacher in the finest sense of the word. He is learned, dramatic, and unbelittling. Perhaps the gentleness and wisdom that come with age allow this man to teach as few are able.
>
> We have all watched an energetic, slight-of-build, elderly gentleman with greying hair stand before us with the implements of colored chalk and a two-dimensional blackboard. With these things at hand, he has created before us a living third dimension of his subject, anatomy. Concomitantly, he has instilled within us comprehension through simplicity: an often neglected approach in teaching medicine.
>
> We have learned from this man the approach to humans as individuals by observing his actions. He may transiently forget a name but he will not forget a student, each is important to him.
>
> We are indebted to Dr. Grant for his direct inspiration of a tradition at our Medical School. It was out of this feeling of indebtedness that Dr. Grant was given a gift four years ago, a gesture that has developed into the traditional Freshman Christmas party for him.

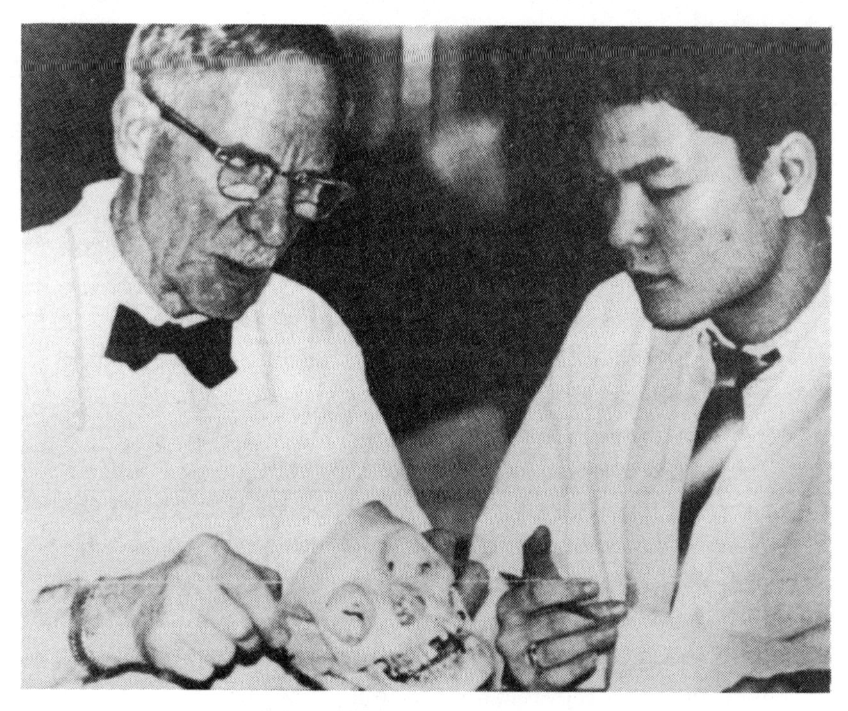

J.C.B. with student at UCLA.

> With these thoughts in mind, the four classes of medical students say: "Thanks, Dr. Grant."

The photograph in the yearbook shows him with glasses, a slight smile and wearing a bow tie and a dark jacket.

May Lesser was one of several medical artists whose talents Grant so often acknowledged. The artists in the *Atlas* are familiar to all who have used it. Grant and Catriona, true to their often spoken gratitude, each made bequests to them in their wills.[2]

The mainspring of her partnership with Grant is explained by Lesser in the introduction to her book:

> This series of drawings and color etchings puts into a pictorial form the highly sensitive human feelings experienced in the process of becoming a physician....
>
> In the first year I shared with [students] the newness and freshness of their approach to the human body, the wonder of the intricacies of the structures, the mood and tension of the anatomy laboratory, and the first impact of the cadaver upon one's sense of immortality.... I shared with them their awkwardness at the bedside when first taking a history, the excitement on the obstetric service....
>
> I had gone to UCLA medical school feeling that studying more structure would be helpful to me. The professor allowed me to audit lectures.... Later he permitted me to come to the Saturday dissection laboratory with the students. At first I was taken aback by the cadavers; the tremendously strong arc lights that were overhead seemed to make the bodies almost transparent in the tank bed.... The students had the rare privilege of having Dr. Grant, who wrote their textbooks on anatomy, lecture to them and help them in the lab. At the age of eighty-three he gave the young people a sense of continuity, a feeling from generation to generation.
>
> He was one of the few MDs with whom the students had contact in the first year.... He tried to teach them some important concept; and so when they left his lecture they came away with an idea... not just notes to be studied later. He would help them picture in their minds relationships in the simplest

form: "Consider the unmatched organs in the abdomen like leaves in a book...."

In his lectures Dr. Grant used his age well: he would ask the students to "help him" recollect some detail! In an era which worships youth, it was pleasant to witness wisdom respected.

Here is a dry-point [May Lesser continues as she refers to one of her illustrations] of him and his assistant professor dissecting out a duodenal hernia in one of the student's cadavers. Although his hands were arthritic, he dissected with blunt tweezers in birdlike movements. In this case he was looking for new specimens for his anatomical museum in Canada.

Dr. Grant had respect for anyone at any level who wanted to learn and he would stay in the lab until the last student finished. When there were no students around, he tried to teach the young woman who worked for him in the embeddding lab... only she argued with him!

A contemporary anatomist of Grant at UCLA, Ebo K. Sauerland, to whom fell the editorship of the *Dissector*, made a visit to Grant's old department in the University of Toronto one year after his death.[3]

I stopped by a nameplate on the door. It read "Dr.J.C.B. Grant". Once inside, the visitor had the strange impression that Dr. Grant had simply left for lunch, temporarily interrupting his work. Grant's white coat was casually thrown over a chair. His teapot and a box of favorite biscuits stood on a shelf. A partly dissected anatomical specimen—several cervical vertebrae, the joint capsules neatly prepared, reposed on a working table. Nearby lay a scalpel, forceps, probe, and magnifying glass. Obviously, the work of the dissector was not quite finished.

A large wall calendar, depicting a beautiful Scottish landscape, showed August 1973. The visitor was jolted to reality. It was now 1974. At the age of 87, Dr. Grant died on August 14, 1973. Only death could end the creativity of this man.

For the past ten years my friendship with Dr. Grant flourished, but thousands of medical students knew Grant only by name. Several generations of physicians learned anatomy by using more than a half million copies of his books, the *Method*, the *Atlas*, and the *Dissector*. Those who studied under Grant never forgot him, while those who never met him desired to know him.

As a teacher, Dr. Grant was exacting in the classroom and laboratory. He so impressed his students, that Anatomy was repeatedly voted the most popular course in the Medical Faculty (quite a feat). At UCLA, the medical students dedicated their yearbook to him. A teacher-evaluation form by the UCLA Student American Medical Association rated him ''A+, a real inspiration to us all.'' Despite seniority and fame, Dr. Grant transcended the boundaries between generations. His mind was fertile; moreover, he radiated a compassion for his fellow beings that students understood and loved.

When I visited the late Dr. Grant's personal and professional environs, I talked with his closest friend and colleague. Only then did I realize the astonishing pattern of coincidence that merged the lives of two scientific giants. Both were sons of ministers and were classmates. Both obtained their medical degrees in 1908 from Edinburgh. After serving as military physicians, both men came singly to Manitoba and subsequently accepted chairs at the University of Toronto. Both became related by marrying sisters, were neighbours in a Toronto suburb, and achieved world recognition through medical writing. Dr. William Boyd, the pathologist, and Dr. J.C. Boileau Grant, the anatomist, are names to be reckoned with!

Grant was not the last anatomist to be called out of retirement to teach at UCLA. Another was R.J. Last who had also written an excellent textbook of anatomy. Last had a longer tenure at UCLA than Grant but he started at a younger age.[4] Grant did not retire as Emeritus Professor at Toronto until 1956 when he was seventy. He was not ''tapped'' for Los Angeles for another five years. He had turned eighty-five by the time he left UCLA—long enough for a working life!

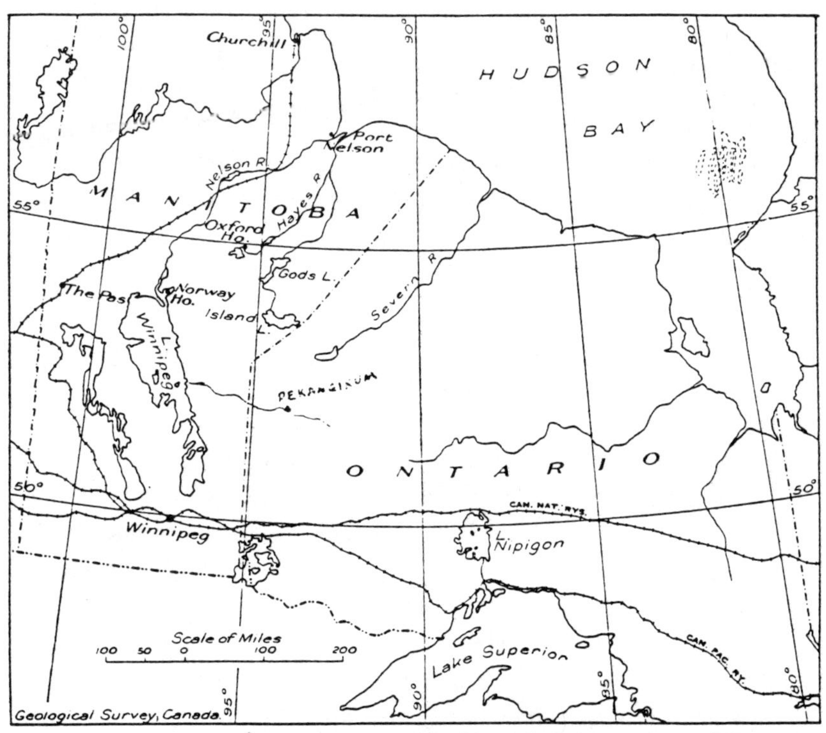

Index map showing positions of Island lake, Gods lake, and Oxford House, northeastern Manitoba.

Map of Manitoba and northern Ontario: areas of first anthropometry of Native peoples (Indian).

— Chapter 9 —

Anthropometry and Other Research

GRANT had his first summer vacation in 1920. After visiting the Mayo Clinic at Rochester, Minnesota, and the University of Minnesota at Minneapolis, he turned north. As medical officer to an Indian treaty party he went by canoe down the Nelson River to York Factory and Port Nelson at the mouth of the river on Hudson Bay, and then turned up the coast to Churchill.[1] When he learned that practically no anthropometric work had been done among the North American Indians of Canada, Grant grasped the opportunity for research before further intermixture with other races (especially Caucasian) could take place. With the help of Diamond Jenness[2] of the Division of Anthropology, former National Museum of Canada, he spent many of the next summers measuring the Indians northeast of Lake Winnipeg, around Lake Athabasca and in the Northwest Territories.[3]

He took with him a variety of instruments: an anthropometer, calipers, a sliding compass and an additional measuring rod; a surveyor's spirit level attached to the measuring rod replaced the original plumb line to ensure that it was held perpendicularly. He also carried a number of common tools unrelated to his researches. Often a Roman Catholic priest accompanied him as interpreter and companion to help with the camping chores.

Grant made about two dozen measurements on each subject studied. Some were complicated. Take, for example, height. Many Indians would not take off their footwear. Some wore moccasins, usually deerskin, some wore thin rubbers over moccasins and some had ordinary rubber lace-up boots. To correct for these variations of footwear he subtracted one millimetre for plain moccasins, about two millimetres for rubbers over moccasins, and three millimetres for pure rubbers. As well as standing height, he measured sitting height. Other measurements included arm stretch length, length and width of hand, and the ratio of index to ring finger length. The condition of the teeth, eye colour, the condition and quality of the hair (baldness was only present in Indians with some European blood), the length and shape of the nose, the upper lip, mouth and ear, and the state of the beard were all meticulously recorded.

The head measurements included the maximum length in the sagittal plane from occiput to glabella, the maximum width (biparietal), width of the forehead (bifrontal minimum), length of the face (both mentor-nasion and mentor-crinion), width of face (bizygomatic maximum), height and width of nose, length of mouth, length and width of ear and length of upper lip.

From these measurements various indices were calculated. The stature index was the ratio of sitting height to standing; cephalic index, the width of head to its length; cephalo-facial index, the width of face to width of head; facial index, the length of face (mentor-nasion) to width of face; nasal index, the width of nose to height of nose; ear index, the width to length of ear; and the hand index, width to length of hand.

On later excursions he took samples of blood for the study of blood groups to be found within the bands. Many populations contained only A, B or O, with no AB group representation.

The little expedition was often regarded with the deepest suspicion and volunteers were sometimes hard to come by. In the years just after World War I, some Indians, fearing that co-operation in what they took to be a census might result in their conscription for a future war, took off into the bush at the sight of the European. Grant learned by experience that the best time to carry out his measurements was on the annual Treaty Day on the reserve when the usual largesse was distributed. A band was then easily accessible and in a less suspicious mood. Children at a Chipewyan orphanage were studied without arousing suspicion or hostility.

Cree and Saulteaux (Ojibway) at Norway House, Oxford House and God's Lake were studied in the early 1920s and the results published in 1929.[3] Some spoke pure Saulteaux, others Cree, while still others spoke a mixture of the two languages. Cree was spoken at Oxford House, a mixture at Island Lake and God's Lake. Migration from further east was responsible for the mixed dialect.

At Island Lake there had in the past been abundant miscegenation with Europeans which was detected in Grant's anthropomorphic observations. He was not, however, able to confirm that the Island Lake Indians had intermarried with Eskimos (Inuit). Local legend had it that, six generations earlier, the Island Lake band had invaded an Eskimo community to the north and brought back the women after murdering the men and children. That this was a fiction was established by Grant's conclusions. It may have been an echo from the past when, 1500 miles to the northwest on 17 July 1771, "Hearne's Chipewyan companions massacred the sleeping Esquimaux Eskimos on the explorer's third journey to find the American Arctic Ocean and a possible North-west Passage."[4]

Grant discovered an interesting marriage custom. While for the most part the practice was common for cousins to marry, they nevertheless adhered to the tradition of not marrying into their own totem. Since a girl on marrying assumes her husband's totem, any children she has may and do marry her brother's children, and in so doing a marriage between different totems is effected. While the children of brothers do not marry each other, brother's children may marry sisters' children with the approval—and arrangement—of the parents. Marriage to a person of another band was of course approved and a number of spouses of each sex were brought into the band in this manner. One extremely old man in this region had two wives.

The long periods men spent away on the hunt may have been the reason for the more liberal conjugal tradition amongst the Inuit. When the Dutchman Willy de Roos was sailing (single-handed) the Northwest Passage in 1977, he saw a woman waving. Not wishing to lose the advantage of a following wind he held his course. A few days later he met an Inuit fisherman who said, "That was my wife; she was likely lonely and you should have stopped and stayed with her."[5]

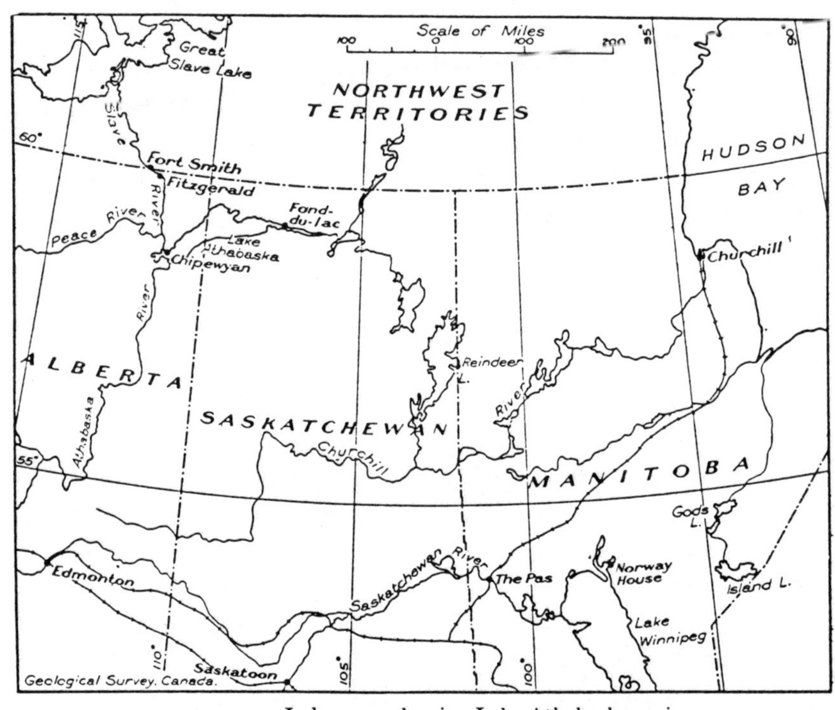

Index map showing Lake Athabaska region.

Map of area of further research around Lake Athabaska.

The excursion the following summer was to Northern Alberta to visit and measure the tribes around and to the north of Lake Athabasca: Fort Chipewyan at the western end, Fond-du-Lac on the east, and Fort Fitzgerald and Fort Smith to the north on the Slave River. The party travelled by train from Edmonton to Fort McMurray, thence by water down the Athabasca River to Fort Chipewyan. The 175 miles along the length of Lake Athabasca to Fond-du-Lac was by motor-driven trading boats. For the separate excursion north, the trading boats were exchanged for canoes to portage the rapids on the Slave River between Fort Fitzgerald and Fort Smith.

From the scientific point of view the expedition was as profitable as it was adventurous. Grant's diary of the trip, in its scientific precision and careful understatement of the hardships endured, has the same authentic ring of the northern explorers of earlier days.

> Forest fires, which had destroyed the country and the timber for a distance of more than 50 miles from the lake shore, a scarcity of fish, and a severe epidemic of influenza at the time of my approach to Fond-du-Lac, did not serve to make my mission popular. Having, in the meantime, fallen in with an Indian agent's party, which likewise was bound for Fond-du-Lac, I attached myself to it. I remained behind at Fond-du-Lac, however, for several days after the party had left, until finding that I should be unable to achieve fully the purpose of my journey. I decided to overtake and join the agent's party, which was now en route for the reserves at Fitzgerald and Fort Smith.
>
> By doing so it seemed probable that I should glean more than by remaining where I was. I, accordingly, made my way to Chipewyan. While awaiting there for the river-boat which would take me to Fitzgerald, I found that almost every Indian had vanished, for their treaty had been paid; but this was not an entire loss to me, because before setting out for Fond-du-Lac I had fortunately delayed long enough to measure them.
>
> To conclude that summer's work, in all 213 Indians were examined; of these, 160 were over twenty years of age. For the most part, they are Chipewyan, but some are Cree and others are breeds. It might be stated that the Chipewyan Indians at Fond-du-Lac might, from the location of their

reserve, be expected to be less mixed (or more pure) than those at Chipewyan and at Fitzgerald and Fort Smith. The coarse quality of the hair of the head and the relative absence of hair on the upper lip, chin, and cheek, and the large percentage of dark-coloured eyes are among the descriptive characters which support this.

The very high percentage of persons with sound teeth, and the small numbers of decayed teeth among those whose teeth were not quite sound, seemed to lend this further support. The distribution of their blood groupings, however, supplies evidence that points in the contrary direction. But the high cephalo-facial index (98.6), especially when considered in connexion with the absolute width of the head and face, of which measurements it is a product, loudly proclaims the Fond-du-Lac band to be much more nearly pure than are the other two.

These Indians have been dealt with first by bands; secondly, those ''assumed to be pure'' Chipewyan have been contrasted with those who are Chipewyan-white breeds. In this second method of grouping, the opinions of the interpreters, which are based on a personal knowledge of the people, were allowed to guide us in making the selection. It becomes evident from a consideration of their general characteristics, teeth, blood, and physical proportions, that those ''assumed to be pure'' are actually slightly more mixed than the Fond-du-Lac band as a whole. As no band of Indians can very well nowadays be totally denied all freedom from white admixture—for in the nature of things some white or partly white persons must be presumed to have married into every band—it follows that the testimony even of informed and well-meaning interpreters is not to be accepted without reservation.

A large percentage of convex noses, a larger percentage of dark eyes, and a larger percentage of persons with sound teeth were seen this year in the northern part of Alberta than last year in the northern part of Manitoba.

The Chipewyan Indians are short in stature; the Cree and Saulteaux measured last year were tall. The similarities in the measurements of the Cree investigated this year at Chipewyan and those last year at Oxford House are, in most cases, surprisingly close. In the few respects in which these two bands of Cree differ from each other they resemble, respectively, neighbouring tribes: the Chipewyan Cree resemble the Fond-du-Lac Chipewyans of Athapascan stock, and the Oxford House Cree resemble the Saulteaux at Island Lake, who, like the Cree, are of Algonquian stock. This may point to the fact that both the Fond-du-Lac Chipewyans and the Chipewyan Cree are more pure than the Oxford House Cree; and that the Island Lake Saulteaux may, moreover, be more mixed with white blood than is supposed. If this be the case, then we are advised as to what physical proportions Indian blood dominates; and what white blood.

Both bands of Cree have finer hair and poorer teeth than the Fond-du-Lac Chipewyans. The blood groups of each of the thirty-three Cree examined belong to Group O (Jansky 1). These Cree, therefore, are universal donors. Whether this is by coincidence or not, further data will reveal.

Somewhat tentatively and on meagre data the males and females of the three great stocks in Canada, namely, Athapascan, Algonquian, and Siouan are compared. It would appear that the most noteworthy difference between the physical proportions of the men of these three stocks is expressed by their cephalo-facial indices, which indices, however, must not be considered without paying due regard to the diameters of the skull from which they are derived.[6]

The similarities in the measurements of the Cree investigated this year at Chipewyan and those last year at Oxford House are, in most cases, surprisingly close. In the few respects in which these two bands of Cree differ from each other they resemble, respectively, neighbouring tribes: the Chipewyan Cree resemble the Fond-du-lac Chipewyans of Athabapascan stock, and the Oxford House Cree resemble the Saulteaux at Island Lake, who, like the Cree, are of Algonquian stock. This may point to the fact that both the Fond-du-lac Chipewyans and the Chipewyan Cree are more pure than the Oxford House Cree; and that the Island Lake Saulteaux may, moreover, be more mixed with white blood than is supposed. If this be the case, then we are advised as to what physical proportions

Indian blood dominates; and what white blood.

The next report[7] was based on observations made in 1929, and includes some work done by Diamond Jenness in 1923 on the Sekani and Carrier Indians. The data on which this report was based is set out in Grant's summary (here edited):

> This report deals with the descriptive characters, measurements, and blood groupings of certain tribes of pure Canadian Indians of Dene or Northern Athapascan stock. These tribes are the Beaver Indians of Peace River; and the Sekani, and Eastern and Western Carrier Indians of Fraser River. The number of adults examined were sixty-four males and forty-two females, in all one hundred and six adult persons. In addition to these a number of old people and children were measured. When to these are added the adult Chipewyan Indians in 1928, the number of pure, or assumedly pure, Dene Indians is brought up to one hundred and seventy-one, of whom one hundred and eight are men, and sixty-three are women.

In this report Grant states that the Beaver tribe was regarded by other Indians as inferior. No member of another band would marry into it. For the Beaver intermarried within families, brother to sister, grandfather to granddaughter. One brother had children by his three sisters. This was obviously more than interbreeding between cousins, even when of a different totem. The skin colouring of the Beaver was darker than the pure Chipewyan. The blood groups were all O or A; none was B or AB. He concludes:

> Of descriptive characters the hair, nose, eye, lips, teeth, digital formula, and blood groups are remarked on; of the sixteen measurements taken twelve are related to the head; the remaining four are stature, sitting height, and length and breadth of hand. The intertribal differences between these Indians are for the most part not great. Notable are the high percentage of eyes of lighter shades among the Carrier and Sekani Indians; and the high percentage of group A blood among the Beaver Indians.

> These people are short in stature, broad headed, with very high cephalo-facial index. For purposes of comparison the measurements of thirty-six Chilcotin men and twenty-two Chilcotin women, a tribe allied to Carrier Indians, measured by Boas and Farrand in 1897, are considered. They are seen to have broad and very short heads, broad and short noses, and a very low cephalo-facial index. This is, of course, surprisingly low (93.3 for men and 91.9 for women), and to be accounted for not by absolute narrowness of the face but by the relatively very great breadth of the head.

Grant applied his deductive skill in his interpretation of an incomplete Inuit skeleton he ''obtained'' (he doesn't reveal details of the circumstances of its acquisition) on the bank of the Churchill River as it empties into Hudson Bay.[8]

> Over a year ago I obtained certain parts of an Eskimo skeleton from the west coast of Hudson Bay, in fact from the left bank of the Churchill River, about four miles above that desolate and once almost impregnable stronghold, Fort Prince of Wales; despite its forty cannon it ''surrendered at discretion'' in the year 1782 to La Perouse.
>
> The parts of the skeleton found were, along with the complete skull, the right sided bones of the upper limb and a right femur.
>
> There is, a little further up the river, a post belonging to the Hudson's Bay Company. To it from time to time the Eskimos from the north bring down their furs; but the territory itself is in possession of the Chipewyan Indians.
>
> The Indians of this neighbourhood differ absolutely from the Eskimo in their method of disposing of their dead, for while these Chipewyans inter theirs, the Eskimo do not, but rather leave them on the surface of the ground, protected commonly from the attack of wild animals by a covering of ice or stones. The bones here described are part of a skeleton which lay extended on the surface of the ground with two long poles covering it, apparently to protect it from the weight of a cairn of heavy stones which was piled over it. Undoubtedly the

entire skeleton lay buried here and it is unfortunate that the bones found were the only ones to be seen.

That they belonged to one who had not been dead for more than a year or two is probable from the fact that the cranial cavity still contained some brain substance and that a slight amount of flesh still adhered to all bones.

Certain points were mentioned to indicate that this was the skeleton of a middle-aged male. ''The articular surfaces at the elbow joint showed advanced osteo-arthritic changes. The surfaces of contact between the humerus and radius were markedly eburnated and the articular margins (humeral, radial and ulnar) of the joint were fringed with 'candle grease drippings'.''[9]

Turning to the skull, one finds that it presents the features which are characteristic of this race, being scaphalocephalic, having the facial aspect of the flat maxilla. The glenoid cavity is deep. The nasal orifice is long and very narrow. Clearly it is an Eskimo skull with a high biparietal-bizygomatic index—probably a full-blooded one at that.

One of the exacting domestic duties of Eskimo children and of the females of all ages is the chewing and biting of the skin of the hairy seal in order to render it supple and pliable that it may be worn as garments. For this reason, the excessive use of the jaws obscures occasionally the customary differentiation of male from female skull.

Coming next to the teeth, we find several features of interest. Certain of them are missing, the absent canines and incisors have no doubt dropped out in the handling of the specimen; but from the degree of alveolar absorption that has taken place, it is evident that several have been lost through disease. The remaining teeth are moderately well worn and bevelled and some are very badly chipped, but there is no suggestion of dental caries.

If the teeth are healthy, with their sockets it is otherwise, for the ravages of pyorrhea alveolaris and of resultant alveolar abscess formation are only too apparent. One would note especially that one abscess cavity, involving the socket of the palatine root of the first right upper molar, has erupted into the maxillary antrum and communicates with it by means of a round hole, 7.0 mm in diameter.

It is generally supposed that prehistoric man was not affected by dental caries and that the same is true of primitive peoples in our own day. Thus, it was stated of a recently discovered Rhodesian skeleton, that "in addition to the traces of abscesses, caries was present in the teeth themselves. This was a condition not hitherto found in any primitive skull." Again, the anatomist Keith in England had observed that "caries of the teeth was a rare disease in Britain until the period of the Roman occupation."

It is therefore doubtful if the present findings contribute anything of moment in regard to the question of caries; but this is the first recorded case in the Eskimo of direct infection of the antrum by extension from a tooth socket.

It is now well known that osteoarthritis, dental caries and alveolar abscesses have been common in Egypt and Nubia even from predynastic times, sometimes occurring together and sometimes not. One research paper on that era described a skull with bilateral antral perforations. These were found in an old woman from the third dynasty cemetery at Tourah "who had upper teeth worn down to stumps and on each side a huge hole near the site of the first molar, communicating with the antrum."

Grant's case, then, with antral perforation, was the first and closest parallel finding in the Eskimo to anything previously recorded.

In 1935 Grant and Storton were the first to excavate an early Iroquois burial site near Brantford in southern Ontario. Many skeletal remains were removed to the Department of Anatomy and were later catalogued by J.E. Anderson and later moved to the Department of Anthropology at Erindale College in the University of Toronto. Grant did not publish the results of his work at the Brantford ossuary, but a recent publication on the recovered bones by Mullen and Hoppa credits Grant and Storton with their discovery.[10]

* * * * *

The subject of duodenal diverticula was one of great and continuing interest to Grant.[11,12,13] The first case he reported he discovered in the dissecting room. There were two diverticula, both in the second part of the duodenum; the larger was 4.2 x 1.8 cm, the smaller 0.73 x 1.7 cm. The larger was 6.0 cm distal to the ampulla of Vater, and the smaller 10.0 cm distal to it. Each seemed to sit astride a bifurcating artery, giving the impression that a herniation of the mucosa had taken place at the bifurcation of a vessel.

The second published case had been found in the dissecting room by a student. (Grant was careful to give him due credit.) It was in a male aged forty-seven, and was situated on the concave side of the second part of the duodenum at the junction of the common orifice of the bile and the pancreatic ducts. It measured 2.5 x 1.2 cm.

The last publication on duodenal diverticula described 15 cases of single or multiple diverticula out of 133 subjects examined in the anatomy department. There were 13 males and 2 females with an age spread from 17 to 80. As Grant said, ''A dissecting room population is perhaps not entirely representative of the population as a whole, but it is at least representative of a certain social class of the community; and the fact that diverticula, whether large or small and whether causing symptoms or not, occur in so considerable a proportion of any section is worthy of attention.''[11]

By injecting the gut with wax before dissection Grant demonstrated the number, shape and position of the diverticula, some of which would otherwise have been overlooked. Most diverticula measured 2.0 cm to 2.5 cm in width, but the dimension of the largest was 8.5 x 3.9 x 5.6 cm. In the article he discusses the theories of causation of duodenal diverticula put forward by other authors without arriving at a firm position himself. Whatever theory he may have favoured, the lack of evidence in support of it prevented him from abandoning his scientific objectivity.

The theme of *applied* anatomy runs throughout Grant's scientific publications. The body's structure had already been revealed in all its details by anatomists of an earlier age. He was not concerned merely to keep that knowledge alive for its own sake. His mission was to use it as a starting point for new concepts in comparative and developmental anthropology and, to the immediate benefit of humanity, as guidance for the hands of future surgeons.

He turned his investigation, amongst other topics, to the anatomy of the synovial membranes which envelope all joints and provide essential lubrication. Their anatomy and function, though understood, had not stirred the attention of anatomists. Grant showed that the layout of the membrane, particularly at major limb joints, could have important practical implications.

"This article," he writes,[14] "with its accompanying illustrations, calls attention to the constancy with which folds of synovial membrane are to be found in healthy and normal joints, to the extraordinary extent to which these folds project between the articular surfaces of bones, and to the fact that they occur at all ages." He continues:

> That fringes and pedunculated outgrowths of synovial membrane lining joint cavities may exist in the pathological state is very well known, but anatomical and surgical textbooks do not furnish adequate indications of the presence of synovial folds in health. References to them are so lacking that it may be doubted if their presence can be generally known or their clinical importance appreciated. They are apt either to be destroyed by the incision which opens the joint or else to be unfolded when the joint capsule is put upon the stretch, and so they elude detection. For their effective display, the tissues of the joint must have been so fixed and hardened that the folds retain both their shape and position when the joint is opened. Once, however, their existence, nature, and positions are appreciated, no difficulty will be found in devising suitable means to display them.
>
> It will be sufficient in the meantime if the existence of these extensive folds be emphasized, for once their existence is known their profound clinical significance becomes apparent. It will not be necessary to do more here than suggest that when a joint is sprained some of its folds are of necessity crushed and bruised, and that the bruising may result in the formation of adhesions, and further that these folds may suffer from various infections as do the valves of the heart.

Illustrations of dissected joints accompany the text to show with great clarity the variations in the anatomy of the synovial folds he encountered, by means of which he alerted surgeons to their clinical significance.

For this and other work at the University of Manitoba, Grant used cadavers on which students, postgraduate and graduate, received instruction and had carried out the dissections. Some specimens had become too dry and others too extensively dissected to be included in the study. But he had convincingly demonstrated that diarthrodial joints, great and small (including the joints of the fingers, toes, hand and foot) contained, at all ages, intra-articular folds which therefore could not have been either acquired or pathological.

In 1925 Grant wrote an article entitled ''On Appreciation of Anatomical Relationships''.[15] It begins: ''It is frequently stated and no doubt frequently believed that 'anatomy is merely a question of memory'. For some reason the other subjects which enter into the medical curriculum are regarded as falling into a different category; a knowledge of them once acquired is retained presumably forever. I would suggest that a knowledge and understanding of anatomical relationships and details depend upon an appreciation of certain principles and facts, and upon logical reasoning, as much as does a knowledge of other medical subjects. These remarks apply to all parts and to every structure of the human body.'' He uses the example of the abdomen to make his point:

> The abdominal cavity contains, first, the gastro-intestinal tract and its derivatives (pancreas, liver and spleen) and, second, three paired glands (adrenal, renal and sex glands). During embryonic life these glands and their ducts lie on the back wall of the abdominal cavity on each side of the vertebral column and covered by the peritoneal membrane. At this early stage of development, the gastro-intestinal canal is a straight tube of uniform calibre, slung from the front of the vertebral column and aorta by a fold of peritoneum, the mesentery. The intestinal canal elongates to about twenty-five feet, and so cannot lie along the middle line of the body. The small intestine becomes convoluted, while the large intestine, taking the superior mesenteric artery as an axis, rotates and encircles the small gut. In the process of taking up their new positions the ascending and descending colon lose their mesentery, but the

> transverse and pelvic segments of the colon retain theirs. Lower down, the rectum retains its position in the midline. During this rotation of the gut, some portion of the small intestine must be crossed by the superior mesenteric vessels. This occurs at its upper end, at the third part of the duodenum.

Grant then describes how the positions within the abdomen of its several organs are inevitably determined by one phenomenon: the rotation of the gut. The position of the few structures not derived from the gut nor directly affected by its rotation are imprinted on the student's mind by the apt simile: ''As did the thread that Theseus trailed after him in the labyrinth indicate to him by what paths he had wended his way, so do the ureters indicate to us the paths of migration of the kidneys, and the deferent ducts and the spermatic vessels the paths of the testes.''

Without burdening the memory it is then easy to understand why the lymph glands which drain the ovary and the testis lie in the lumbar region, whereas those which drain the scrotum and labia majora are situated in the groin. These are matters for appreciation, not for memory.

He points out that the veins draining the gastro-intestinal tract must also drain the pancreas and the spleen since they are gastro-intestinal offshoots. It then follows that venous drainage from the adrenal gland or kidney cannot join the gastro-intestinal drainage since they arise from morphologically separate systems. To confuse the two, he says, is to treat a hot water system as one with the electric light.

Thus he stresses the value of a knowledge of embryology in relieving the student of an overburdened memory. The migratory movements of structures during intrauterine growth lends a rationality to the apparently haphazard and asymmetrical placement of thoracic and abdominal contents.

His texts and classroom teaching were illuminated with scraps of extraneous information and references to daily life that fixed anatomical facts effortlessly in the mind. The sphincter that separates the mouth of the fish from the stomach is the analogue of the human oesophagus, a tube created as the diaphragm descended. Fascia, the inelastic membrane which covers most muscles, is not to be found in the anterior abdominal wall. If it were, he points out, we would look forward to

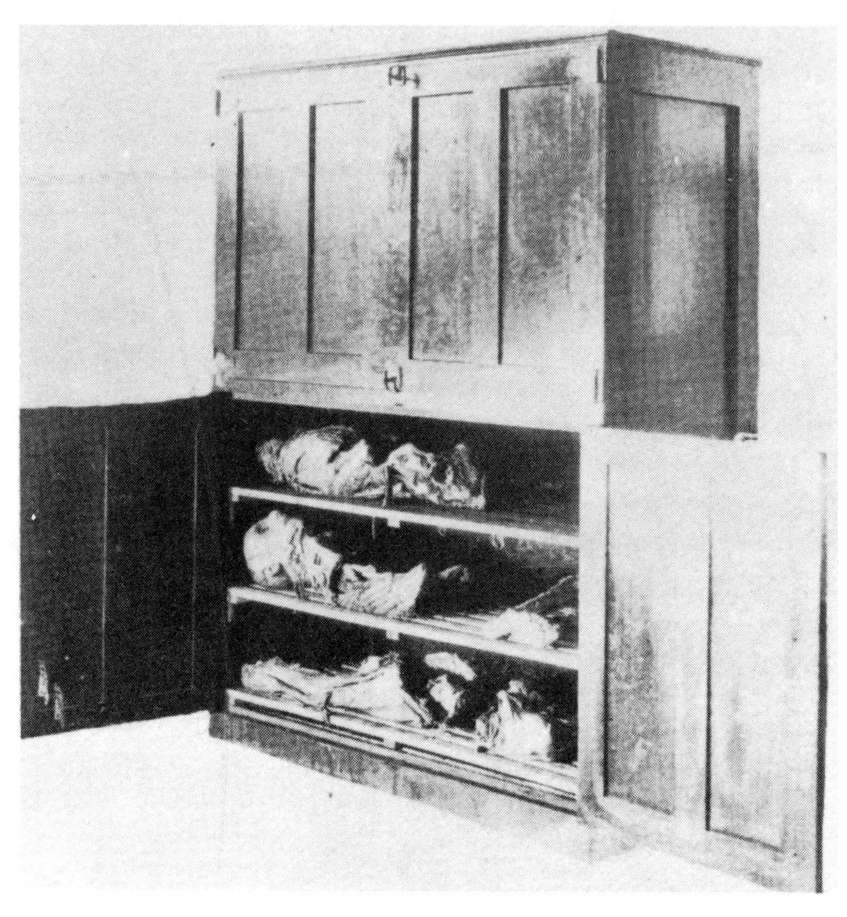

Storage cabinet for anatomical specimens. (Anat. Record 34:91-93, 1926)

the next meal with apprehension rather than pleasure, and abdominal respiration would be impossible. The flat cells which lie on a loose membrane and with it constitute the peritoneum, are no more ''the peritoneum'' than wallpaper is ''the wall''.

A somewhat unexpected but highly practical article appeared in *Anatomical Record* of 1926 entitled, ''Storage cabinet for anatomical specimens''.[16] In it Grant describes, with a photograph, a structure made from wood by the carpenter at the University of Manitoba. It was 70½ inches in height, 50½ inches in width, and 27 inches deep. It was, of course, an upright cabinet; there were six shelves, each nearly 18 inches apart, so that an arm or a leg could be conveniently accommodated. A removable, galvanized pan, fitted on the floor immediately beneath the bottom shelf, contained a preservative fluid which supplied sufficient vapour to keep the specimens moist and in good condition. The cabinet had two pairs of well-fitted, hinged doors.

It was designed to replace the usual metal-lined tank of the day, constructed after the fashion of a travelling trunk, with lid and tray. Storage was wasteful of floor space, and the specimens below the tray were not accessible until the tray and its contents had been lifted out. Grant's new wooden cabinet held as many specimens as three of the old tanks, and occupied the floor space of only one. Also, as it rested on four casters, it could be wheeled easily from one room to another.

— Chapter 10 —

Honours and Awards

WILLIAMS and Wilkins, the publishers of Grant's very successful first *Method of Anatomy,* were so impressed on seeing his museum at the medical school in Toronto that they urged him to produce what became the *Atlas of Anatomy,* the second of the three books published by Williams and Wilkins and the first anatomical *atlas* to be published on the North American continent.[1]

Grant was elected second Vice-President of the American Association of Anatomists for 1950-1952. He considered his election as honorary president of the Canadian Association of Anatomists in 1956 (which, of course, lasted for the rest of his life) an even greater honour.

He received an illuminated parchment from the Officers of the American Association of Anatomists at their annual banquet in 1957, held that year in Baltimore. In celebration of the unique occasion the citation read:

> Because of his great contribution to the teaching of human anatomy on this continent, and his furthering of the happy relations of American and Canadian anatomists for nearly forty years, this Citation is awarded by the Executive Committee of the American Association of Anatomists to Dr. J.C.B. Grant,

Professor and head for many years, of the Department of Anatomy of the University of Toronto, Canada.

Edward A. Boyden President

Louis B. Flexner Secretary

Presented this seventeenth day of April, Nineteen Hundred and Fifty-seven, Baltimore, Maryland.

The following year at a special convocation on 10 October 1958 the University of Manitoba conferred on Grant the degree of Doctor of Science (honoris causa). Dean Bell, presenting Dr. Grant to the Chancellor, said:

Mr. Chancellor, I have the honour to present JOHN CHARLES BOILEAU GRANT, Bachelor of Medicine, Bachelor of Surgery, Fellow of the Royal College of Surgeons of Edinburgh.

Doctor Grant was born a son of the manse, near Edinburgh, attended school in Edinburgh and Nottingham, and graduated in medicine from the University of Edinburgh in 1908.

True to the Edinburgh tradition, Doctor Grant chose anatomy as his career, and demonstrated Anatomy at the University of Edinburgh and the University of Durham. His career was interrupted by the First World War, in which he served as a medical officer from 1914 to 1919. For meritorious service he was mentioned in dispatches and was awarded the Military Cross.

In 1919 he was invited to apply for the Chair of Anatomy at the University of Manitoba, a post previously held by his great friend and classmate, the late Dr. Alexander Gibson. During his eleven years in this Faculty, Dr. Grant proved himself to be one of the greatest living anatomists. His method of anatomy, later incorporated into a textbook, was a vivid and unforgettable exposition of a difficult subject. His interest in anomalies and in anthropology lent further distinction to his teaching and writing. His return to this school has illustrated again the great affection all his former students felt for Dr. Grant as a teacher and friend.

Dr. Grant accepted the Chair of Anatomy at the University of Toronto in 1930 and held that post until his retirement in 1956. He has, however, continued to act as curator of the anatomical museum.

When the Canadian Association of Anatomists was founded in 1956, Professor Grant was elected honorary president *sine die*. This was official recognition of his position as doyen of Canadian anatomists.

On behalf of the Senate of the University of Manitoba, it is my privilege to request that you confer upon John Charles Boileau Grant, Bachelor of Medicine, Bachelor of Surgery, Fellow of the Royal College of Surgeons of Edinburgh, the degree: Doctor of Science *honoris causa*.

Of all Grant's professional colleagues the hardest hit by his death were, perhaps, his Toronto staff members Ross MacKenzie and J.S.Thompson. Their regard for him during his life and dismay at his death reflected the admiration of so many who, in or out of the classroom or laboratory, counted him their friend. MacKenzie and Thompson, in their eulogy, said:

...Dr. Grant was not only an author of distinction. Year after year his class in human anatomy was voted by the students as the most popular in the faculty and the memory of him as a teacher burns so brightly that in 1973 the class of 1948, at its 25th reunion, presented him with a plaque in appreciation for his teaching example and stimulation....

His actual contributions can, of course, never be totally assessed. Many, who never met him, spoke his name with a touch of awe. Those who knew him may visualize his amazing energy as, even long after his retirement, he bounded up the stairs two at a time to reach the library to check a point of fact or confirm an authorship. Others may recall the enthusiam with which he prepared specimens, many of which became the nucleus of the museum which now bears his name. His knowledge of anatomical fact was encyclopedic and he enjoyed nothing better than sharing his knowledge with others whether they were junior students or senior staff. While somewhat strict as a teacher, his quiet wit and boundless humanity never failed to impress. He was, in the very finest sense, a scholar and a gentleman.

Chapter 11

Triumph, Finale

JOHN Charles Boileau Grant died on Tuesday, 14 August 1973. His death was noticed by many Canadian newspapers and by the *New York Times*. The influence he had had over the thousands of medical students who had passed through his hands, many later becoming eminent surgeons and physicians, was acknowledged in the obituaries, as well as his work in criminology through identification and the ''reading'' of human bones.

In his early period at the University of Toronto, he refused to sit for a portrait. But after he became Professor Emeritus, Dr. John Basmajian persuaded him to have it done. Cleeve Horne's portrait, commissioned by Grant's former demonstrators, now hangs in the anatomy department.

The illustrious career of John V. Basmajian included an association with Grant as student and staff member at Toronto; later he became head of the Department of Anatomy at Queen's University, Kingston. Basmajian had a strong attachment to Grant, a mixture of father-son and teacher-student relationships. Of Grant he wrote at his death:[1]

> For the host of his admirers and students around the world, news of Dr. Grant's death brought an overwhelming mixture of sadness, nostalgia and grateful reminiscences. His long and fruitful life was devoted to service to others. The users of his books are numbered in the hundreds of thousands in many lands, and several thousands of Canadian physicians and surgeons were the direct recipients of his generous efforts.
>
> For six decades he was a magnificent classroom teacher. From his start as a demonstator of anatomy at Edinburgh until his second "retirement" at age 85 from his perennial visiting professorship at the University of California in Los Angeles, only four years took him away from students. These were the years of the 1914-1918 World War. Not that he ever mentioned these facts. Such matters would make him acutely embarrassed. Indeed, when the "MC" after his name was misrepresented as a minor surgical degree, he would not bother to correct the error.

While Grant was a demonstrator at the medical school at the University of Durham he came under the spell, at a distance, of the great Professor Elliot Smith, head of the anatomy department at Manchester. There are similarities in the careers and personalities of the two men. Besides his teaching skills in topographic anatomy, Elliot Smith was a distinguished neurological and comparative anatomist, anthropologist and archaeologist. He assisted on occasions in criminal investigations, and the British Museum consulted him for the identification of specimens of bone. He was one of the group involved in investigating the authenticity of Piltdown Man, a forgery that apparently deceived Sir Arthur Keith. Elliot Smith, like Grant, was quiet-mannered and reserved, unlike Keith, his more flamboyant rival. Through his own similar nature Grant would have felt an affinity for Elliot Smith and, by his scientific achievements, Elliot Smith would have been Grant's exemplar for his future journeys in Northern Manitoba in pursuit of anthropological discoveries.

Basmajian continues:

> Dr. Grant's heroes were all intensely hard-working and productive people with high ethical motives; not a few were

Edinburgh medical graduates such as John and William Hunter, the immortal Scottish anatomist-surgeons. Most were dedicated medical scientists, but he always admired courage, dedication and wisdom in anyone.

Returning from the war as a major, Dr. Grant did not remain long in Britain. A warm invitation to head the Anatomy Department in the University of Manitoba in 1919 brought him to Winnipeg which was then starting on its amazing growth and maturity. Eleven years later, the bigger, older and wealthier University of Toronto beckoned.

Recently the site of the discovery of insulin and competing for the finest minds, Toronto set out to get the best young anatomist in Canada to succeed the distinguished J. Playfair McMurrich as head of anatomy. The pressure was great and persistent, but Dr. Grant had established an outstanding anatomy laboratory in Manitoba that was difficult to leave. In addition, his physical anthropology research with Northern Canadian Indians had become a consuming interest.

Yet a greater duty called, and in 1930 he moved to Toronto where his career as a great teacher and author of textbooks began to achieve its finest expression. Although anthropometry remained an important aspect of his anatomical interests, he never again had the opportunity of travelling among the northern tribes about whom he had written several definitive monographs.

His textbook *A Method of Anatomy, Descriptive and Deductive* was the natural outgrowth of his deductive lectures and demonstrations, conceived and perfected at Manitoba and finally published in 1937 in Toronto. Those of us who had the privilege of using his books and studying anatomy with him are convinced that our heritage is unique. This includes many thousands of medical graduates, but all-too-few anatomists. Among the hundreds of postgraduates he trained, only a handful were planning careers in anatomy.

Constantly revising, improving and perfecting the accuracy and expressiveness of every line in the *Method,* Dr. Grant brought it to a dominant position. It was not until he had completed and published the sixth edition in 1958 that he felt he could entrust the burden of future editions to another. Curricular changes have dictated changes of emphasis in the five editions that have appeared since then, but the deductive reasoning that was the benchmark of his teaching remains unchanged and enduring.

While the *Method of Anatomy* was helping to reform teaching in the English-speaking world, his even more popular work appeared and was hailed during World War II. Grant's *Atlas of Anatomy,* first published in 1943 and since appearing in a long series of revised editions, soon became the world's most widely used anatomical atlas. Only those who have helped in its preparation know how meticulously it was prepared, what exquisite pains were taken in the accuracy of the dissections and drawings, how carefully everything was checked and rechecked. The reader only sees the beauty and clarity that is apparent to even a layman. Behind them is craftsmanship of unbelievable quality.

Officially Dr. Grant retired as head of anatomy in Toronto in 1956, but this only removed the need for his supervising a department. As Professor Emeritus he accepted the responsibility of Curator of the Anatomy Museum—which is now named after him in its new quarters in the magnificent Medical Science Building of the University of Toronto. Every specimen bears the imprint of his work.

Soon after his retirement, the University of California at Los Angeles discovered that he had spare time on his hands during the winters. And so began his second career as a visiting professor in the early 1960s. In that role he made many more new friends among students who recognized the unique nature of his teaching in the laboratory. Perhaps the only times I glimpsed his open pride of personal accomplishment was when he would tell me (not without considerable amazement) of the expressions of affection and gifts given by students at UCLA. In 1970, the administration of UCLA could no longer ignore the fact that their visiting professor was some twenty years beyond the retirement age for everyone else, and Dr. Grant gave up active student contact. But his energetic work in Toronto continued with his beloved *Atlas* and museum over

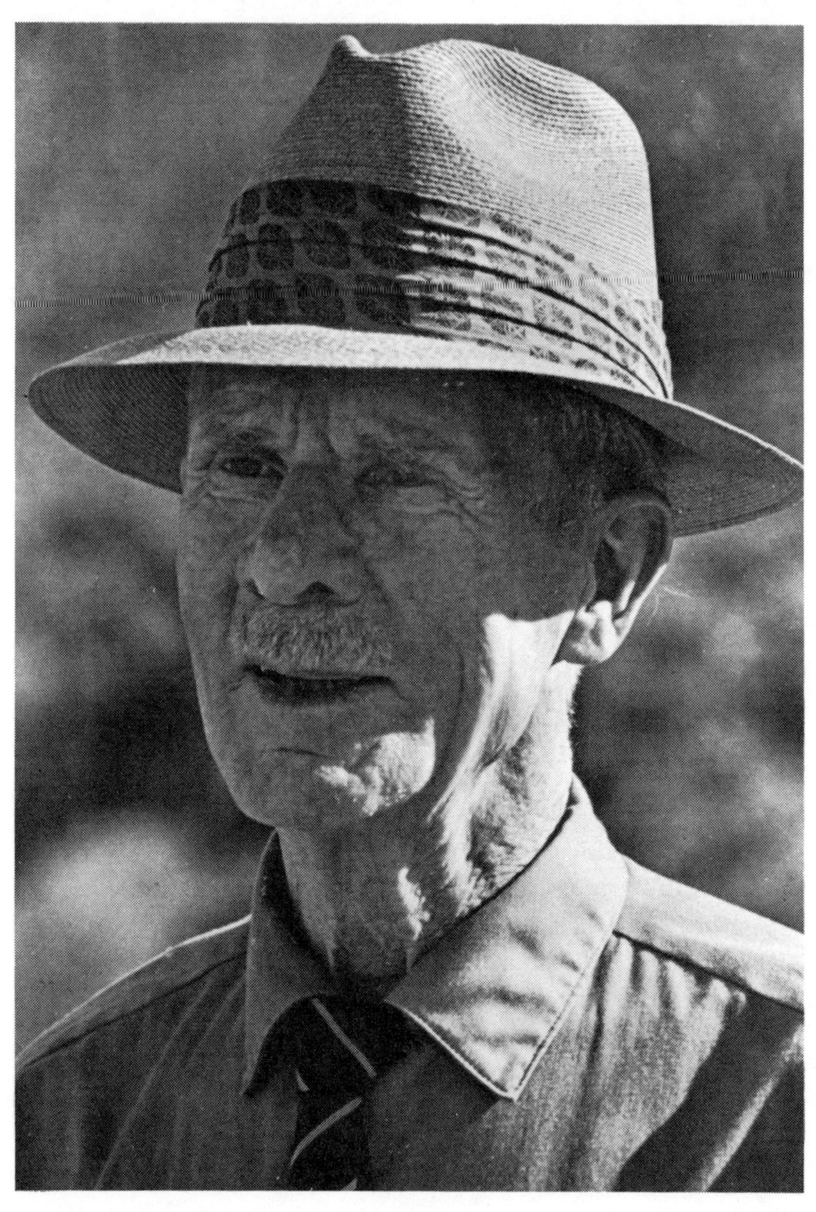

J.C.B.

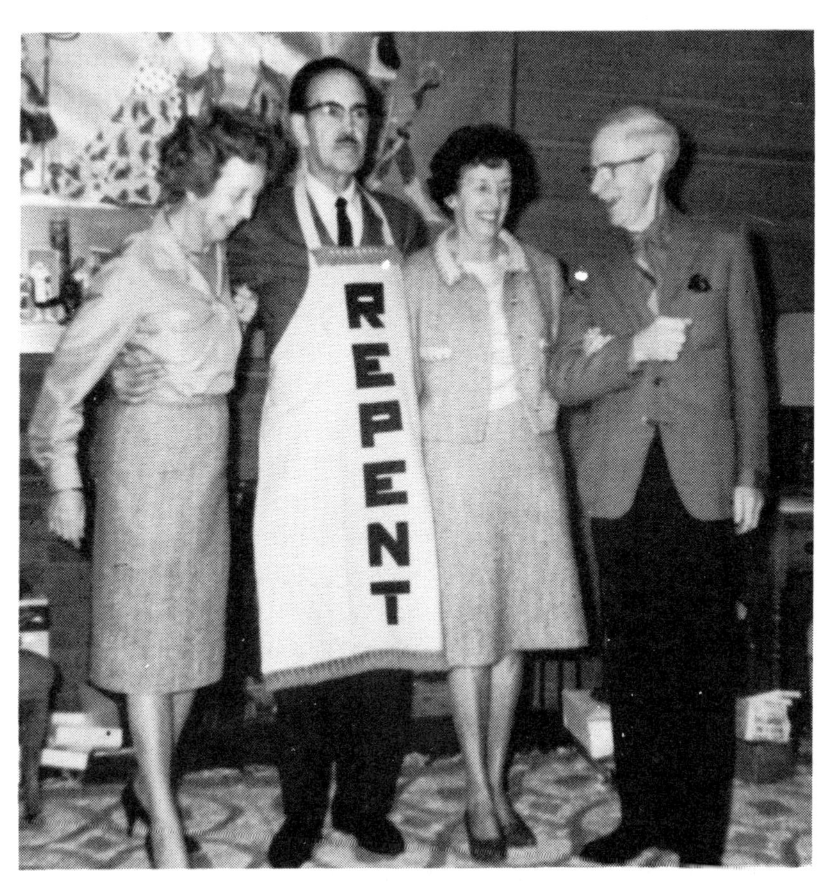

Christmas, 1964, Portland, Oregon, at the Feir home. Mary (Christie) Feir, Dr. David Christie, Catriona, and J.C.B.

the remaining three years.

He was also a long-time member of the Anatomical Society of Great Britain and Ireland.

An erudite, sparkling, indefatigable man, Dr. Grant had a warm and soft side that came out in private. With his wife Catriona by his side, his wit and charm were infectious. Catriona, whom he met and wed in Manitoba, was the great pride of his life, perhaps the only pride he showed without embarassment; and she reciprocated in a way that was a pleasure for all of us around them. Her loss is immense, for rarely are two persons so much like one. While they had no children, many of his students and colleagues will remember Dr. Grant just as they do their real parents. His other children, his books, will speak for us and keep his name alive for many generations.

In correspondence with me John Basmajian enlarged upon the reasons for his admiration for his mentor:

The facts of his career in medical schools were easier for him to discuss with me and this he did quite freely as part of my education—because it involved his teachers and role models rather than himself. One aspect masked by Dr. Grant's painful modesty was a paradoxical and white-hot pride in his scientific accomplishments and his family connections. He successfully shielded the world from his conviction that there were (in the world) a huge mass of *plebes* and a tiny minority of creative and brilliant people that he was sure he (and I!) belonged to. Thus his low regard for the former group was sometimes painful, and for the latter it expressed itself with a fine sense of admiration of leading heroes on the one hand and a regard for "noblesse oblige" on the other.

One of the reasons that Dr. Grant never enjoyed or sought a personal camaraderie amongst professional anatomists had nothing to do with modesty. (He was openly proud of the world-wide success of his books while he sought the shadows.) The reason was that he trained very few anatomists. I believe it is correct that I am the only one whom he recruited, while Jim Anderson was recruited by me and later (just near his retirement) by Dr. Grant.[2] Other distinguished anatomists could count dozens of their students who became senior professors. When I raised money to have Dr. Grant's portrait painted, some 150 surgeons were traced who had been demonstrators with him—but I do not recall a single PhD whom he had trained.

Of course, this reflects Dr. Grant's conviction that gross anatomy is part of surgery. That attitude did not make him friends among anatomists in North America. Today, as that profession is admitting, clinical anatomy is critically important in medical education. Fortunately Canadian clinicians recognized then and now that Grant was a giant in applied anatomy. As I wrote in his obituary, he remains the greatest teacher of human anatomy in the English language since John Hunter.

I suggested to John Basmajian that Grant's excessive pride was not a virtue and might even be considered a fault. He said in his reply of 2 November 1989: "Your point re a great man's disabilities or warts is valid. Certainly well-concealed pride is not a great failing; in some people, open pride bordering on arrogance is deemed a virtue. But remember, my remarks are from an adopted son who well may have talked about deeply personal matters (his as well as mine)...."

Grant faced death with composure. He knew he had a serious cancer but had no fear of the inevitable. His "intelligent agnosticism", as his nephew Ian Reid characterized the extent of his religious belief, was a modification of his youthful Presbyterian indoctrination. It carried him quietly out of his life as harmoniously as it had supported him in it.

On the plinth of the engraving in the *Fabrica* of the erect skeleton in pensive posture, Vesalius has inscribed

Vivitur ingenio, caetera mortis erunt.

Genius is too strong a characterization of Grant, but his spirit and his influence will surely live when others have passed into oblivion.

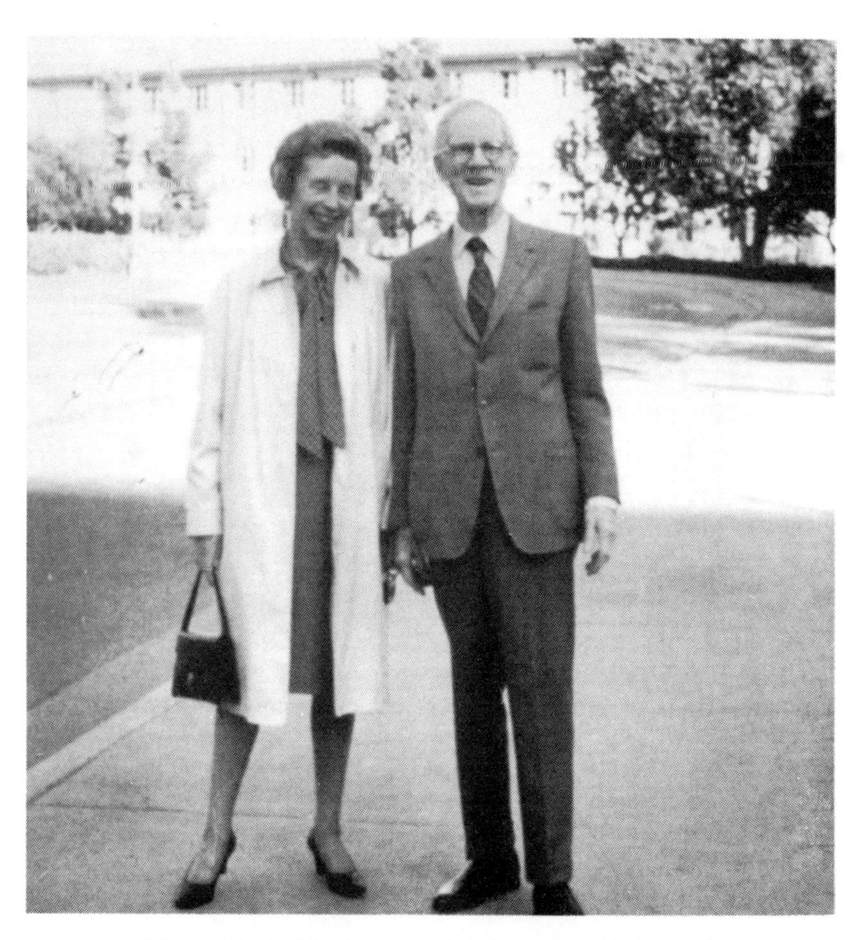

Mary (Christie) Feir and J.C.B. at UCLA in 1969.

Notes

Acknowledgements

1. Robinson, C.L.N. Further remembrances of that revered anatomist Dr. J.C. Boileau Grant, *Can. J. Surg. 31*: 203-204,1988.

Chapter 1

1. Hay, David. *Whitehaven: An Illustrated History*. Whitehaven: Michael Moon, 1979.
2. Muriel, G.J. *A Short History of the Whitehaven and West Cumberland Infirmary 1783—1924* (revised by T.E. Woodhouse and G.G. Carter). Whitehaven: W. H. Moss and Son Ltd., 1924.

Chapter 2

1. Loanhead. *Groome's Gazeteer*, 1895. (Courtesy of Dr. W.P. Small, Edinburgh.)
2. Rev. Grant's unpublished reminiscences, ***A Humble Human***, are in the custody of his grandson, Ian Reid.
3. Further unpublished material, courtesy of Ian Reid.
4. Grantown-on-Spey. *Groome's Gazeteer*, 1895. (Courtesy of Dr. W.P. Small, Edinburgh.)

Chapter 4

1. Leacock, Stephen. *Our British Empire*. London: John Lane, Bodley Head, 1940. Chapter 4, p.140.

Chapter 5

1. Cornford, F. MacDonald. *The Republic of Plato*. London: Oxford University Press, 1941. p.160.

Chapter 6

1. Grant wrote his *curriculum vitae* a few years before his death. At the time of the journeys, Diamond Jenness had not yet been admitted as Companion of the Order of Canada (CC), the highest civil honour, limited to 150 living members.
2. Appendix I. Refs. 7,9,14.
3. Boyd, W. Cause and Effect. The 5th Alexander Gibson Lecture. *Can. Med. Assoc. J. 92*:868-869, 1965.
4. *High River Times*. High River, Alberta. 20 June 1963.
5. Appendix I. Ref. 15.
6. Appendix I. Ref. 6.
7. Persaud, T.V.N. A brief history of anatomy at the University of Manitoba. *Anatomischer Anzeiger* (Jena), *153*:3-31, 1983.

Chapter 7

1. MacKenzie, R.G. *A History of the Department of Anatomy of the University of Toronto*. Unpublished. University of Toronto Archives. The account covers the years 1824-1973.
2. Smith, C.G. *Basic Neuroanatomy*. Toronto: University of Toronto Press, 1961. (2nd edition 1971)

I first met Carl Smith when he had been appointed to the Algerine Escort, *HMCS Middlesex*, in Halifax. He was senior to me by a half stripe (Surg. Lt. Commander to my lowly Surg. Lieut.). His quiet modesty concealed from me his distinguished career in anatomy, and it was not until I joined Grant's department as a demonstrator that I discovered his other, civilian persona. He had shed his uniform but his meticulous attention to the task in hand and his politeness to his juniors had not changed.

3. Kalkman, J.W. Personal communication.
4. Bell-Irving, P. Personal communication.
5. Harris, W.R. Professor, orthopaedic surgery, University of Toronto.
6. Doll, R. and Bradford Hill, A. A study of the aeteology of cancer of the lung. *Brit. Med. J.* 2:1271-1286, 1952.
7. Elliott, A.J. Professor of Ophthalmology, University of British Columbia. Personal Communication.
8. The Lord Stanley whom Grant rescued and who opened the Canadian National Exhibition at Toronto in 1936 died in 1938 at the age of 44. His father, the 16th Earl of Derby, who outlived him, was Governor General of Canada (1888 to 1893). He donated the Stanley Cup for hockey and Stanley Park in Vancouver was named after him.

Chapter 8

1. Lesser, May H. *The Art of Learning Medicine*. Englewood Cliffs, N.J.: Appleton Century-Crofts, 1974. Preface.
2. The artists for the *Atlas* were Dorothy Chubb, Nancy Joy and Eila Hopper Ross.
3. Sauerland, E.B. Anatomist extraordinaire. *J. Amer. Med. Assoc.* 232: 1347-1348, 1975.
4. R.J. Last, Australian born, as a young surgeon was torpedoed in the early days of the World War II while returning home from London. He was rescued and taken back to England where he took up an appointment as professor of anatomy at the Royal College of Surgeons — which had recently examined him for the surgical specialty diploma, the fellowship. He stayed at the Royal College for the whole of his working life and there he wrote his anatomy textbook. When he retired he returned to his native Australia and it was there that he was asked to accept a visiting professorship at UCLA. He continued at UCLA for another seventeen years until his second retirement in Malta, where, a widower, he lived in a Roman Catholic retirement mission home. He died there on New Year's Day 1993.

Chapter 9

1. Grant does not dwell much on the trials and hazards of his northern travels. According to his own record it appears that he visited Churchill on the same trip that took him to Port Nelson, which would have meant turning north at Port Nelson up the shore of Hudson Bay for 240 km. The flat, windswept shore is inhospitable for canoe travellers and is made doubly dangerous by the extensive muddy shallows impassable on foot. The canoes may have been driven by small (but cumbersome by modern standards) outboard motors to buck the prevailing northwesterly wind. The other possibility is that he made a second trip down the Churchill River to the port of Churchill, which was the usual route of access from the hinterland.
2. The late Diamond Jenness was created Companion of the Order of Canada in 1969 for his anthropological work among the aboriginal people of Canada. The first of numerous editions of his classic, *The Indians of Canada*, was published in 1932 as Bulletin 65 of the National Museum of Canada.
3. Grant, J.C.Boileau. *Anthropometry of the Cree and Saulteaux Indians of Northeastern Manitoba*. Ottawa: National Museum of Canada Bulletin no.59:1-73, 1929.
4. *The Coppermine River*. A wild river survey descriptive report. Ottawa. National Parks Service Planning Division. 10-28 July 1972.
5. de Roos, Willy. *Vancouver Sun*, 9 June 1978. p.17. He sailed the Northwest Passage single-handed.
6. Grant, J.C.B. *Anthropometry of the Chipewayan and Cree Indians of the neighbourhood of Lake Athabaska*. Ottawa: National Museum of Canada Bulletin 64:1-31, 1930.
7. Idem. *Anthropometry of the Beaver, Sekani, and Carrier Indians*. Ottawa: National Museum of Canada Bulletin 81: 1-17, 1936.
8. Idem. Some notes on an Eskimo skeleton. *Amer. J. Phys. Anthrop*: 5:267-271, 1922.
9. The likeness to candle-grease drippings refers to the appearance, not the texture, of bony incrustations at the edge of the joints, similar to changes which had been described by Léri and Joanny (Léri, A. and Joanny J. Une affectation non décrite des os; hyperostose "en coulée" sur toute la longueur d'un membre ou "mélorhéostose." *Bull. Med. Soc. Hop.* Paris 46:1141. 1922), except

that Grant's description applies to the common joint-related hyperostoses rather than the shaft of long bones.
10. Mullen, G.J. and Hopper, R.D. Rogers ossuary (AgHb-131): an early Ontario Iroquois burial feature from Brantford Township. *Can.J. Archeol. 16*;32-47, 1992.
11. Grant, J.C.B. Duodenal diverticula. *J.Anat. 57*:357-359, 1923.
12. Idem. On the frequency and incidence of duodenal diverticula. *Canad. Med. Assoc. J. 33*:258-262, 1935.
13. Idem. An anomalous duodenal pouch. *Brit J. Surg. 23*:233-234, 1935.
14. Idem. Interarticular synovial folds. *Brit. J. Surg. 18*:636-644, 1930.
15. Idem. On appreciation of anatomical relationships. *Canad. Med. Assoc. J. 15*:1195-1201, 1925.
16. Idem. Storage cabinet for anatomical specimens. *Anat. Rec. 34*:91-93, 1926.

Chapter 10

1. MacKenzie, Ross G. *A History of the Department of Anatomy of the University of Toronto*. Unpublished. Archives, University of Toronto. 48 pp.

Chapter 11

1. Basmajian, John. Dr. J.C.B. Grant. Obituary. *Anat. Rec. 180*:176-178, 1973.
2. Anderson, James. Taught anatomy in Toronto under Dr. Grant in the 1960s. Dr. Grant passed on his interest in anthropology to Anderson who moved to the Department of Anthropology at the State University of New York at Buffalo. When the new medical school at McMaster University in Hamilton, Ontario, was being organized he was appointed Professor and Chairman of its anatomy department. Anderson confirms that Grant saw his role more as an educator of aspiring surgeons than of future academic anatomists.

Appendix 2

1. Agnew, D.C.A. *Protestant Exiles from France in the Reign of Louis XIV*; also Huguenot Refugees and Their Descendants in Great Britain and Ireland. Edinburgh and London. 1866.

The first edition was privately published; the second edition was corrected and enlarged, was given an index, and appeared 1871—1874; the third edition (1886) was greatly enlarged. All editions were published by Reeve and Turner. The third edition included the history of French-speaking refugees in foreign regions and was for ''private circulation''.

Most of the information and some (edited) passages on the Boileau family are taken from Agnew, vol. 3. p.213 et seq., 3rd edition, and some are taken from vol. 1.

2. *Les Métiers et Corporations de la ville de Paris, XIIIe Siècle*. Imprimerie Nationale. Paris: René de les Pinasse et François Bonnardot. 1879.

—— Appendix I ——

Publications of J.C.B. Grant

1. Grant, J. C. Boileau. Some notes on an Eskimo Skeleton. *Am. J. Phys. Anthropol.* 5:267-271 , 1922.
2. Idem. Duodenal diverticula. *J. Anat. 57*: 357-359, 1923.
3. Idem. On the appreciation of anatomical relationships. *Can. Med. Assoc. J. 15*: 1195-1201, 1925.
4. Idem. The significance of a skull. *Quart. J. Univ. N. Dakota 16*: 106-122, 1926.
5. Idem. Storage cabinet for anatomical specimens. *Anat. Rec. 34*: 91-93, 1926.
6. Idem. Teaching anatomy at the University of Manitoba. *Bull. Assoc. Amer. Med. Coll.* 3: 1-10, 1928.
7. Idem. *Anthropometry of the Cree and Saulteaux Indians in Northeastern Manitoba*. Ottawa: National Museum of Canada Bulletin 59: 1-73, 1929.
8. Idem. Interarticular synovial folds. *Brit. J. Surg. 18*: 636-640, 1930.
9. Idem. *Anthropometry of the Chipewyan and Cree Indians of the neighbourhood of Lake Athabaska*. Ottawa: National Museum of Canada Bulletin 64: 1-31, 1930.
10. Idem. The learning of anatomy. *Med. J.* (Univ Toronto) *8*: 123-128, 1931.

11. Idem. *Progress in an anthropometric survey of the Canadian aborigines.* Fifth Pacific Science Congress. June 1933.
12. Idem. An anomalous duodenal pouch. *Brit. J. Surg. 23*: 233-234, 1935.
13. Idem. On the frequency and incidence of duodenal diverticula. *Can. Med. Assoc. J. 33*: 258-262, 1935.
14. Idem. *Anthropometry of the Beaver, Sekani, and Carrier Indians.* Ottawa: National Museum of Canada Bulletin 81: 1-17. 1936.
15. Idem. *A Method of Anatomy, Descriptive and Deductive.* Baltimore: Williams & Wilkins Co., 1937. (11th Edition, John Basmajian and Charles Slonecker, eds., 1989)
16. *Grant's Dissector.* (A Handbook for Dissectors). J.C.Boileau Grant and H.A.Cates. Baltimore: Williams and Wilkins Co., 1940. (9th Edition, E.K. Sauerland, ed., 1984)
17. *Grant's Atlas of Anatomy.* Baltimore: Williams and Wilkins Co., 1943. (10th Edition, Anne Agur, ed., 1991)
18. Idem. The dissections of the synovial tendon sheaths in the hand and foot, illustrated in the English edition of *Gray's Anatomy*, 29th Ed., London: Longmans, Green & Co., 1946.
19. Idem. Respiratory system in Cunningham's *Textbook Of Anatomy*, 9th Ed., London: Oxford University Press, 1951.
20. Idem. Muscular system in Morris's *Textbook Of Anatomy*, 11th Ed., Toronto: Blakiston Co., 1953, with the assistance of Carlton G. Smith.
21. Idem. *A Method of Anatomy.*
    Indian Edition, Calcutta, in English.
    Italian Edition.
    Japanese Edition.
    Chinese Edition, in English.
22. Idem. *Atlas of Anatomy.*
    Japanese Edition, Igaku Shoin Ltd., Tokyo.
    Spanish Edition, Inter-Medica SAICA, Buenos Aires.
    Italian Edition, Intermedical, Rome.
    Indian Edition, S. Chand & Co., New Delhi. In English.

— Appendix 2 —

Boileau Ancestry[1]

Part of the Boileau ancestry is recorded here because Grant was so proud of it. He usually insisted for official purposes he should be styled ''J.C.Boileau Grant''. His pride in the Boileau connection may have owed something to a common sense of chivalry in battle and duty through his dedication to service to his students. I have selected a few of the more distinguished forebears for mention.

Family of Boileau, Lords of Castelnau de la Garde and of Saint Croix de Boyreac.

The family of Boileau has the most magnificent pedigree of any of the refugee (Huguenot) families. Etienne Boileau, Grand Provost of Paris in 1255, was an historical personage, and the pedigree traced back to him is without a flaw or gap. The family was ennobled in 1371.

Etienne Boileau (1205— ?)

Etienne married Marguerite de la Guèle in 1225. His family had originally come from Orléans; he had been mayor there before moving to Paris.

In 1248 he went on the seventh crusade led by King Louis IX (St.

Louis). He was captured with the prince in 1250. He regained his liberty by paying a ransom of 200 pieces of gold. To procure that considerable sum he leased for 10 pounds of gold per year a house he owned in Paris near the church of Saint Germain-l'Auxerrois.

Etienne's father was *Mathieu Boileau* (then spelled Boilesve); he died in 1251 and was buried near the Abbey of Saint-Euverte.

The prince, St. Louis, made Etienne the Mayor of Paris after their return from the crusade. Etienne had a reputation for modesty and humility, leaving few records by his own pen of himself.

The Book of the Trades[2] describes the legacy he left to Paris. The statutes he promulgated survived for five centuries as the legal code for the settlement of contentious issues between private and corporate parties. He advanced the commercial interests of the city by organizing many trades including flour mills, groceries, drapery and clothing stores, potteries and their products. For the social welfare of the community he promoted legal services, medical specialties, and apprenticeships. He established a police force, reformed the justice system and codified penalties for malefactors.

The Boileau line after Etienne was represented by many prominent citizens—good reason for Grant to be proud of his ancestors.

Robert Boileau, who died in 1277, had been a Crusader.

Jean was ennobled by Charles V (The Wise) by letters of nobility registered in Paris in 1371. Messire Jean was killed in the battle of Nicopolis (1369) when the Christians were defeated by the forces of Bagaget, Emperor of the Turks.

Noble *Regnaud*—Treasurer to the King's dominions of the Seneschalship of Beaucaire and Nîmes, in the province of Languedoc, 1390, died in 1400. He was the first of the family to live in Languedoc; before this he lived at Montereau-faut-Yonne where he had a house, still standing, which he sold for 4500 livres. Charles VI erected a castle at Nîmes in Lower Languedoc which the Boileau family incorporated into its coat of arms. Later, Etienne's grandson came to live at Nîmes and took the crescent into his arms to commemorate the family's participation in the crusades.

Noble *Guillaume*—Treasurer of the domain in the Seneschalship of Beaucaire and Nîmes. His receipts were derived from the Bishoprics of Nîmes, Montpellier, Uzès and Mindevivière and forty-three ports from Frontignan on the Mediterranean coast to Lyons on the Rhône.

In 1492 Charles VIII settled the patronage of the office on Guillaume and his son. In 1470 he married Estiennette Bourdine, daughter of Jean Bourdine, General in the King's army at Poitou. Her dowry was 400 gold crowns. Guillaume died 6 September 1491. His tomb is in the house of his descendants at Nîmes. He fathered eleven children, the eldest of whom was Antoine.

Noble *Antoine*—He inherited his father's official duties. He bought the lands and jurisdiction of Castelnau de la Garde and of Saint Croix de Boyreac in 1500 from the Secondine of St. Felix. He married the daughter of Noble François Trossellier, Physician to the King. Antoine died in Italy on his return from Naples, leaving four children.

Noble *Jacques Boileau*—Lord of Castelnau etc. (1626—1697) married Frances de Vignolles, with a dowry of 20,000 livres. When the Edict of Nantes was revoked and Frances no longer could enjoy its protection, she was confined first in the Convent of Payeu and then in the Convent of the Ursulines at Nîmes from which she fled to Lyons. Two years later (1690) she escaped to Geneva, later joining her family in Brandenburg.

In 1652, Jacques Boileau, being of the reformed church, was chosen to represent the opposition to the Bishop. For his defection from Rome he was imprisoned in 1687, with several others, in the Château de Pierre Excise at Lyons. He became ''paralytic'' in 1696 and died at the age of seventy-one on 17 July 1697 after a captivity of ten years. Of his 16 children, several died in infancy. Of the others, some fought for the reformed church while one, *Maurice* (b. 1678), remained in France and kept on the Boileau name by recanting to save the estates. That Maurice's recantation was inspired by a hard-headed decision to hang on to the family property is further suggested by his naming his three eldest sons after their uncles Henry (1665—1709) and Jean (1667-1733), who were killed serving under the Elector of Brandenburg in the Protestant cause, and Charles who survived into retirement in Southampton.

The record of the French line ends in Nîmes in 1811 as the Scottish (Clarke) line joins the Boileau with the marriage of Dr. James Clarke to Harriet Ann Boileau in the first part of the nineteenth century.

Index